MORE SUCCESS STORIES FROM THE STAY-AND-SUPPORT METHOD

'Working with Lucy has honestly changed our household . . . I thought I had a baby who just wasn't able to sleep through the night . . . he now goes to bed at 7 p.m. and sleeps right through until 7 a.m. I have so much more energy to play with him and enjoy him and he is a lot happier in himself.'

'By the time we called Lucy, we were zombies! Her advice is so practical – she lifted us out of the fog of sleeplessness! We saw an improvement every few days with our daughter and she now sleeps until almost 6 a.m. without waking, which to us is a miracle!'

'We never thought we'd get a decent night's sleep as our baby and toddler were both waking on numerous occasions throughout the night . . . with Lucy's help our baby went from very broken sleep to sleeping through the night within a week. Our toddler also now settles quickly and easily and sleeps through the night. We would highly recommend Lucy to any parents struggling with sleep problems.'

'Lucy taught us how to sleep train our baby in a very gentle way. We now have a two-year-old who mostly sleeps 11–12 hours a night, and if she wakes she is able to go back to sleep unaided without us having to get out of bed. Be assured that with Lucy you get results!'

'Previously, our night routine was a constant effort to try to get our baby to sleep, and even then he woke every two hours, leading to a fully sleep-deprived family. Now, he is sleeping 12 hours a night, knows how to fall asleep by himself, enjoys the routine and wakes happy and relaxed. We saw major results from the first week of the process. We would highly recommend Lucy and her methods.'

'Our baby would wake for three to four hours during the night, keeping us all awake. Now he goes to bed between 7 and 7.30 p.m. and sleeps until about 7 a.m. I can't tell you how amazing that is. It's still such a great feeling to get a full night's sleep, even months later!'

LUCY WOLFE is a paediatric sleep consultant and mum of four children. She is the head of Sleep Matters, where she has many years' experience and a proven track record in helping babies and children learn to sleep more soundly. She has completed extensive training, certification and continuous professional development with the Gentle Sleep Program (USA), with further studies in Child Sleep Consultancy, Postnatal Depression and Child Nutrition, accredited by the OCN (UK). She has specific training and certification for children aged four to five months, with continued studies in Parent Mentoring and Relationship Studies (UCC). She is the former European Director of the Association of Professional Sleep Consultants and a member of the International Association of Child Sleep Consultants. Lucy is a regular contributor to RTÉ and TV3 television shows on the subject of sleep, as well as various radio shows and print and online publications including the Irish Independent, Mums & Tots, Maternity & Infant and Mummypages.ie. For more information visit www.sleepmatters.ie.

THE
baby sleep
SOLUTiON

The stay-and-support method to help
your baby sleep through the night

LUCY WOLFE

First published in Ireland in 2017
by GILL BOOKS
Gill Books is an imprint of M.H. Gill and Co.

First published in Great Britain in 2019
by Headline Home, an imprint of
HEADLINE PUBLISHING GROUP

8

Cataloguing in Publication Data is available from the British Library

ISBN: 9781472269157

HEADLINE PUBLISHING GROUP
An Hachette UK Company
Carmelite House
50 Victoria Embankment
London EC4Y 0DZ

www.headline.co.uk
www.hachette.co.uk

I would firstly like to thank my husband Alan for his love, support and unwavering belief which has made all of this possible. To my children Jesse, Ellen, Eden and Harry, who each in their own way provided very fertile ground for learning and understanding the challenges around childhood sleep. Thank you for your understanding during the writing process and for the notes left on my desk and bedside locker reminding me to write! Thank you to my parents, who have always believed in and encouraged me.

To the team at Gill Books, much gratitude for understanding that this was a great idea! For your ongoing support and limitless patience – you are all amazing.

Finally, a sincere thank you to all of the parents who have asked for my help – for allowing me the privileged position of entering your lives, putting your faith in me and the process, and being open to direction and guidance, especially when times were tough. To those of you who recommend me at your baby classes, coffee mornings, online and at the school gate – none of this would have been possible without your goodwill. The pleasure has been all mine and the great sleep is yours to keep.

Contents

Introduction

It's good to meet you; it will be my pleasure to help you work through your child's sleep issues in a positive and gentle way. My name is Lucy Wolfe and I am a sleep consultant and mum of four children. When my eldest son was born I knew very little about anything child-related – what was there to know and how hard could it *really* be? Jesse was what some might call a textbook baby; he fed and slept well initially, but as time went on his sleep deteriorated and by 10 months of age he was waking multiple times and drinking his own body weight in milk. I found myself frustrated, confused, challenged and, of course, extremely tired. I couldn't understand how this had happened – he had slept for eight to ten hours from six weeks of age! I desperately needed things to change – for his sake, as well as my own.

I often joke that my career path was changed when I received this call from the land of sleep deprivation. My interest in sleep – the science and the strategies – was spiked by my own sleepless child. After working through *my* challenges and then, when I had three more children, realising that they were all so different and that there are gentle and emotionally considerate ways to help promote better sleep, I decided that I would extend my education and retrain in order to help others.

I work with families and children from birth to six years of age to establish positive sleep associations in the early days and to address frustrating sleep problems from six months onwards – without leaving a child alone to cry. To date I have helped over four thousand families directly and many more indirectly. Now it's your turn.

I want to help empower you to address your child's sleep issues, without compromising your own parental beliefs, with complete respect for your child's emotional well-being and individuality. My approach is distinctly different from many others. First, I absolutely do not advocate unattended cry-intensive methods, controlled crying or crying it out, and I never want parents to leave their child upset in an effort to improve sleep. I suggest that positive sleep practices can be achieved and maintained, safely and appropriately, with a parent-led and fully attended, emotionally attached approach – and I will show you how. It is imperative that your young child feels loved, safe and secure at all times and that lack of sleep does not hold them back developmentally, emotionally or physically. Sleep serves a vital function, and sleep deprivation in early childhood causes an increased risk of health issues, impaired mood and behaviour, low concentration levels, reduced motivation and poorer academic performance.

I have a holistic approach that takes account of all the influences on sleep and merges them together in order to minimise stress and allow the child to be open to learning a new skill, while their natural body clock is in sync. I will always encourage you to attend and support your child, to be instinctive and not to second-guess yourself. My emphasis is on having all the positive sleep components accurately aligned, so that better sleep practices for your family have room to emerge and so that it feels right for you. My work is not about unrealistic expectations about sleeping through the night before your child is biologically ready or crying alone or about trying to drop nighttime feeds when they are still needed; it's rather about setting the scene for improved sleep practices in your family unit so that everyone can function at their optimum level.

No family sets out to experience a debilitating sleep issue and not all sleep-related issues require fixing. However, *all* sleep can be enhanced and improved on and a solid framework can be laid; and you don't need to cry it out to make this happen. The issues you experience can emerge at any age and stage. There will always be contributory factors, which I will help you identify. All children can be encouraged to sleep better. If you can develop a greater understanding of sleep itself and of your child's temperament, and see the connections between the elements that contribute to the majority of child sleep issues, you will be able to help.

A feeling of failure can engulf the sleepless parent – a sense that they have done something wrong, that they *should* be able to sort out the problems without assistance. But all children are different, and what suits one particular child may not suit another. We change as parents, too – I know that as I had more children my own philosophies adjusted. This may be as a result of the changing family dynamic and each child's temperament. We need to make decisions that suit everyone. I happily shared the bed with my youngest child, Harry, as it worked for us – but it may not be what you want and it definitely would not have suited my daughters Ellen and Eden. This book will highlight the reasons why you may be struggling, help you to become informed and aware, and help you to establish positive sleep associations and create the correct sleep environment for your child. It will also help you to develop an age-relevant balance between feeding and sleeping – and along the way it will illustrate common practices that help support and consolidate sleep and provide solutions for the issues with a consistent and clear approach.

Of course, we won't just focus on problems. I will also help the new and expectant family work towards gently shaping their child's sleep from the early days, while at the same time allowing the parent–child relationship to blossom. This can be achieved without being a slave to adult-oriented routines. When we understand how baby sleep actually works, we don't need to be too concerned about what some may call 'bad habits'.

I encourage you to think of your baby and child's sleep in two parts: before six months and after six months. In the early days, your child's sleep is not organised biologically and your baby may have a high need of parental input. I would never endorse a sleep learning exercise in the early days, but I can show you how to meet the baby's needs in the early months and in turn work towards constructive sleep practices for your family so that you never have to troubleshoot. I call this gentle sleep shaping and if you are in the early stages of parenthood or haven't had your baby yet, you might want to skip straight to Chapter 4 to get an idea of my strategies in the early months. Remember to move to the appropriate chapter as your newborn grows, though, so that you continue to create the correct balance for your child's sleep as they transition through the stages. We know that the more informed parents are, the fewer problems they will have with their child's sleep.

If your child is aged between six months and two and a half years of age and you are struggling, we can introduce a sleep learning exercise with my personalised stay-and-support approach, pulling all the influencing factors together to reverse a negative sleeping cycle, while remaining emotionally engaged and allowing your child to achieve their optimum sleep ability. I deal with this age group in Chapter 5, to help you understand sleep in a simple, practical way and then learn to implement my proven, effective approach. It takes time to establish great sleep patterns, so you will need to be patient and confident as you proceed through the stages.

I am also well aware that sleep problems are not just reserved for babies and toddlers. Many sleep issues continue into or emerge in the older age range and come with their own set of challenges – being able to protest, bargain, stall and, of course, run away from you, refusing to stay in bed, insisting that you stay and also sharing their or your bed with you overnight. So I have included a special chapter on how to package up the process and approach for your older child, too, without resorting to reward charts or incentives. In Chapter 6, I attempt to establish children's best practice sleep habits organically and with their co-operation. The key is to provide your child with a sense of ownership and get them invested in their own 'sleep happiness'. You provide choices and a sense of autonomy, but you remain in control, diminishing any anxieties about being alone at bedtime or through the night and consolidating their nighttime sleep, so that they get the rest they need and take great sleep habits into adolescence and adulthood. Older child sleep issues are sometimes brushed under the carpet, with fatigued parents resigning themselves to this being just the way it is; the child is 'just a bad sleeper'. Let's not rest on that premise; let's be proactive and believe. Everyone can learn to sleep better and with confidence, they just need to be programmed correctly. Don't rely on the assumption that your child will grow out of it. It can happen, but it might not.

So let's get started!

Chapter 1

Why Your Child Won't Sleep

First of all, it's important to emphasise that not all sleep challenges require intervention or 'fixing'. Infant sleep is highly complex and not at all organised and so what feels like a problem may well be just what your child's sleep looks like at this early stage. I get lots of messages from worried parents that their two-week-old baby wants to be held and won't stay asleep. This can be hard for the parents, but it is a very natural presentation from someone so young, who has been carried in the womb until so recently and whose whole system is immature. However, as time evolves and your child gets older and more robust, most sleep challenges will benefit from adjustments and intervention. Achieving better sleep for your child and family unit does not need to be about unrealistic expectations, sessions of unattended hysterical crying or trying to drop nighttime feed practices before a child is developmentally ready. It *is* about laying a solid framework for positive sleep practices, without compromising your child's well-being – in fact, we will be enhancing it.

Common sleep issues from six months onwards may be represented by a resistance to sleep (taking up to three hours to go to sleep at bedtime); going to sleep with ease, then waking on multiple occasions, sometimes 8–10 times in a two- or three-hour period; or perhaps staying awake for three hours during the night, waking at four a.m., fighting daytime sleep and taking short and varied naps during the day. You may experience some or even all of the above at various stages. If you are, please know that this is the beginning of the end of the frustration and stress.

From around six months of age, the character of your child's sleep has locked into place neurologically and the originally disorganised nature of infant sleep starts to become more organised. At this stage it more or less looks like adult sleep, except the young child needs more sleep than an adult and they dream more, too. Essentially, your child will start to have to cycle through their natural sleep phases and this is where issues can start to arise. It is not unusual for a 'dream' or 'textbook' baby to start getting more restless. Equally, you may find that issues that began at birth become even worse at around six months. This often coincides with what is referred to as the 'six months regression' and I suggest from this age onwards is the time to really actively start work on sleep issues. I want you to become informed and to gain a greater understanding of why your baby doesn't sleep. Your younger baby will benefit from my gentle sleep-shaping recommendations outlined in Chapter 4, while acknowledging that before six months we don't consider that there are any sleep problems, just an immature sleep state that may need to be actively addressed at a later stage – and it is never too late!

Typical dependencies

There are two major contributory factors to most sleep issues in babies aged six months and over. The first might be described as a parental dependency in the context of your child's sleep. This means that if you are involved in getting your child asleep or partially asleep, your child is not yet independently able to go to sleep themselves. This in turn may mean that they are less likely to be able to cycle through their natural nighttime and daytime sleep phases. In the early months I encourage you to support your baby's needs as outlined in Chapter 4 and I also suggest that you enable your child's sleep ability with the 'percentage of wakefulness' approach. There is a small window of opportunity for introducing this approach, and if you have not been successful to date, the way your child achieves their sleep now can start to be part of a sleep problem. It can seem contradictory because your child needed support from you to get to this point, but now your support can almost go into reverse and represent one of the reasons behind continued sleep issues.

Common levels of dependency for achieving and maintaining sleep include a need for one or more of the following:

- bottles
- nursing
- parental presence
- buggy
- car
- rocker chair
- dummy
- parents' bed
- holding
- hand-holding
- rubbing
- couch

Lucy Says

Needing parental input to sleep beyond six months increases the risk of nighttime activity!

By the age of six months your child's sleep has started to become organised, so if your child is helped to sleep, their brain can find it difficult to maintain sleep duration without further parental intervention. When a child of six months and older who has been helped to sleep starts to cycle through sleep, the brain will periodically have a 'partial arousal'. This is a bit like a 'check-in' system, where the brain checks to see if everything's okay – 'Is everything the same as it was when I first went to sleep?' If it is, your child will more than likely roll over into their next phase of sleep, unless they are hungry and require a feed.

Unfortunately, if there is a level of dependency at this age and stage, when the brain checks in and things are not the same – the bottle/dummy/nipple/parent is no longer present – or the child has been transferred to the cot or bed already asleep or very sleepy, this partial arousal becomes a complete arousal and your child will call, cry and look for you to help them into their next phase of sleep. This dependency leaves you more exposed to unnecessary nighttime activity than you will be with a child who has been able to perfect the skill set. It is not unusual for some children to have been great at sleeping only for things to start to unravel when your initial sleep support stops working.

It is not uncommon for a six-month-old to initially fall into a relatively deep sleep, and you may not hear from them for the first two to four hours after bedtime. But then they awaken. This sometimes coincides with parents going to bed, and they may believe that they have caused this disturbance, but it is generally the end of the first sleep cycle. After this first awakening, your child will generally go into a light, dreamy sleep. You may find that your child wakes more frequently – every hour, every two hours, every 50 minutes, every 20 minutes – and unfortunately each time the child needs your assistance to go on to the next sleep cycle.

Lucy Says

You may also find that as the night wears on, it becomes more challenging to get your child to go back to sleep – what worked at 11 p.m. and 2 a.m. is not as effective at 3 a.m. and 4 a.m. and you may need to work harder or add to your attempts to help your child return to sleep.

By the time we get to 5 a.m. young children want to do one of two things: to get up and start the day; or to go into another deep section of sleep for another hour or two until morning time proper.

When I meet with parents for the first time, at this point they are nodding and laughing, telling me I am describing *their* night (and possibly yours) so accurately that I must know what I'm talking about! You may find that your nights are different from this, or that they vary from night to night, or there is frequent waking directly after bedtime (this links with the second part of sleep issues, which I will outline later).

What I'm describing is essentially the biology of your child's sleep – we can't change that. But we can address the associations your child has with going to sleep and going back to sleep.

Often a dependency is not apparent to parents. It may take the form of a feed that happens too close to sleep time but doesn't put your child to sleep, or it may involve an innocuous re-tuck of the blanket or kiss on the forehead; or perhaps you are still at an initial stage of my 'percentage of wakefulness' approach (described in more detail in Chapter 4). Either way, if your night sounds a little bit like what I have described above and your baby is six months or older, you can rest assured that you are close to the beginning of the end of your current sleep issues.

I call this a partial dependency. It's very often triggered by a feed that happens too close to sleep time – it doesn't put the baby to sleep, but it does help their brain get into a sleepy state. Although many sleep professionals promote bath, bottle and bed, I am keen to change the order and create a greater distance between feeds and sleep to prevent this dynamic interfering with your child's sleep ability. If the feed is much less than 45 minutes before sleep time, I consider it to be part of the problem. I recommend a feed at least 45 minutes before sleep time and entirely separate from the bedtime routine.

Biological timekeeping

The second part of many sleep struggles, and one that is more significant for some families, is all about the internal body clock – your child's circadian rhythm. This rhythm will not be completely set until after the age of around four years, but it is of enormous significance from birth. Your child needs lots of sleep, including daytime sleep, and they also have what I would describe as an ideal time or optimum time to be awake and an optimum time to be asleep. Young children who are not in sync with these times may find it more difficult to either go to sleep or stay asleep or, for some, a bit of both.

Timing for sleep is everything and although in the early days I endorse flexibility, at this age I would perhaps become more prescriptive. Often families that I work with have timing issues and nothing else. This makes the sleep issues no less challenging, but they can often be the reason why parents feel they have 'tried everything' and nothing has worked. If timing for sleep is not addressed correctly, then all the sleep learning techniques – shush, pat; pick up, put down; cry it out – that you may have read about will have limited results. Having a routine is simply not always enough – not all routines are equal – and I would encourage you to look at my age-relevant suggestions outlined in Chapter 9: I know they are effective.

What does your child do when they start to get tired? Perhaps they get cranky, whiney, fussy, moany? These obvious signals usually indicate an overtired child: intense eye rubbing; wide yawns; stretching limbs; clenching fists; arching the back; becoming agitated, a little bit impatient, unreasonable and non-compliant; wanting to get up with you, then wanting to get down again; not really knowing what they want. Or perhaps you don't observe any of these symptoms; perhaps they get a bit hyper, or even a little bit entertaining. Maybe they request familiar items for sleep – their dummy, their lovey, your breast. If you see any of these signs, either in isolation or in combination, your child is highly likely to be overtired. Perhaps you even wait for these signs, because you know that achieving sleep will be easier.

Lucy Says

Allowing your child to become obviously tired means that you are probably in a danger zone. If you see these signals, your child's body is overtired. The body's chemical response to becoming overtired is to secrete cortisol and adrenalin into the system. This has two main effects: it makes it hard to go to sleep, which is why parents find that their child fights or resists sleep; and it also makes it difficult to stay asleep, which further exacerbates frequent nighttime awakenings.

Going to sleep when you are overtired often means that the brain is in a heightened state of neurological arousal. This means that your child sleeps lightly and everything wakes them – a flush of the toilet, creaking stairs, for example. You may be experiencing frequent nighttime arousals directly after bedtime, or maybe long wakeful periods overnight, perhaps some early rising and/or short and varied nap durations. All of this can be a sign that your child's naps or bedtime, or both, are happening when they are already overtired. Sometimes it can be as little as 10 minutes too late!

Understanding 'getting tired'

We have now established what the signs of *being* overtired are. Now let's clarify what *getting* tired looks like.

The signs are not particularly noticeable – I would be looking for a quick eye rub, a brief yawn, maybe a moment of quiet – zoning out, staring into space – momentary decreased activity. Do you see this? Parents often see these signs but they disregard or misinterpret them, generally waiting until the signs are more obvious – which is the point at which your child is overtired.

These signs indicate sleep readiness – your child's body is getting ready for sleep. The hormones, the chemicals in the brain, the body temperature dropping all play a part. The good news is that, given the skill set – we will work on this – and the opportunity that we will start to create, your child could start to go to sleep with ease and stay asleep for as long as their body needs.

Lucy Says

Early sleep cues are a brief eye rub, yawn or moment of quiet. These signpost the ideal time for sleep.

What if you don't see the signs?

It's not unusual for parents to be puzzled and report that they don't see these signs, and that is okay. It doesn't necessarily mean that you are missing the sleep cues. Sleep-deprived children are great at disguising the early signs, leaving you only with the late cues. You may have twins or older children who act as a stimulant, ensuring that you are fooled into always attempting sleep when your child is overtired. Some easy-going babies are also very good at disguising how they feel. Parents often comment during the sleep learning process that *now* they really see the signs – how could they have missed them before? But perhaps they didn't miss them; they just weren't clear. As your child gets better at sleeping, they start to want you to know when the right time is and the early sleep cues emerge and become obvious.

Lucy Says

Some children are great at disguising their early sleep signals.

Others will be stimulated by an older child and also mislead you.

Other have a mild temperament and becoming overtired doesn't seem to affect them, but it does impact on their sleep.

Whether or not you can see these signs, I am going to help you plan an age-appropriate feeding and sleeping structure for your child, with or without sleep cues, that will start to match their biological clock and rhythm. This can help you start to work on improving their sleep, whether or not they give you clues.

Common sleep issues

Symptom	Cause(s)
Wakes frequently overnight	Overtired from nap deprivation
	Parent-dependent at bedtime
	Bedtime too late
	Parent-dependent overnight
Takes ages to get to sleep at bedtime and may or may not wake thereafter	Nap deprivation
	Bedtime too late
	Bottle/nurse/television too close to sleep time
	Nap imbalance
Goes to sleep very easily but wakes frequently	May go to sleep easily due to inadequate day sleep
	Bottle/nurse may be too close to sleep time
	Parent-dependent at bedtime
	Parent-dependent overnight
	Nap imbalance during the day
	Naps attempted at the wrong time
	Bedtime starts too late
Will only go back to sleep with a bottle	Bottle-dependent at bedtime
	Historic bottle dependency at bedtime
	Bottle-dependent overnight
	Negative feeding cycle
	Naps attempted at the wrong time
	Bedtime starts too late
Will only go back to sleep in your bed – may still wake frequently	Your child may go to sleep at bedtime in your arms/bed and is transferred to the cot already asleep and wants out as they awaken
	Naps attempted at the wrong time
	Bedtime starts too late

Will only go back to sleep with a bottle and coming into bed	Bottle is probably used close to bedtime and may be in arms or on parents' bed when they first go to sleep
	Child has expectation of bed-sharing/conditioned hunger from habitual night feeds
	Naps attempted at the wrong time
	Bedtime starts too late
Wakes at 4–5 a.m. to start the day	Bedtime may be too late
	Nap deprivation
	Nap imbalance
	Uses a sleep prop – bottle, parents' presence at bedtime
	Parent-dependent overnight
Naps infrequently	Irregular daytime schedule
	Oversleeps in morning
	Misses sleep window
	Day sleep not prioritised
	Unable to sleep without a dependency at bedtime
Takes 20–30 minute short naps	Overtired from broken nighttime sleep
	Oversleeps in morning
	Naps attempted when already overtired
	Parent-dependent at bedtime, nap time or both
Naps well but still wakes at night Wakes within first hour of bedtime	Nap timing may not be in sync
	Naps may not be balanced
	May require a prop at bedtime
	Bedtime may be too late

Routines

Many parents do not want to be routine-based with their children, and I am aware of all the arguments for and against. I do encourage a feeding and sleep structure from early on, though, and if you have been very flexible to date and are now having sleep issues with your child, adding regularity to your days will have an immediate positive effect on their sleeping pattern.

Of course, many parents are already routine-oriented and still sleep is elusive. I must point out that *all routines are not equal* and you may well have a routine that doesn't suit your child.

Lucy Says

Even with a structured day, if the timings are not aligned with your child's natural rhythm the sleep challenges have a tendency to continue.

Also, if your child has difficulty maintaining sleep or they are always close to being overtired, they are in a weaker position than a well-rested child and the timings need to be adjusted and refined further, which I will help you to do.

In the following pages I will help you:

- establish the best time to start working on your sleep
- make appropriate decisions
- establish positive supports for better sleep
- outline my effective stay-and-support sleep learning approach.

Additionally, I will help you:

- learn how to create your child's age-relevant daytime feeding and sleeping routine
- plan your approach for overnight
- address your daytime sleep issues.

The result?

Better sleep for the entire family.

Chapter 2

Getting Started

Although I appreciate that there is no 'right time' and there will always be barriers to prevent you making changes, I believe that you need to commit to the process so that you make it as easy as possible for your child to develop their new skill set.

1. Ensure that they are 100% well. Take your baby to your GP for a review and get the green light to begin a sleep improvement plan. You don't want to begin this process when your child is sick. Of course they may become unwell at any time, and we can set out a response plan for dealing with this, but only begin when your child is completely healthy.

2. Although your child will be teething on and off now for another one or two years, don't start when they are chronically teething: wait for a gap and then begin.

3. More important, don't start when your child is due to have vaccinations during your sleep learning exercise. Although many children are unaffected by jabs, many can feel under the weather, have pain, develop a temperature, be off form, and some may develop a cold within 10 days, so choose your time wisely, even if they have been unaffected in the past.

Wait for four or five days after vaccinations before you begin a sleep learning exercise.

4. You will need to prioritise your child's sleep for the next three to four weeks. It takes the brain this long to learn a new pattern of behaviour. During this time it is not recommended to go away for the weekend, have a sleepover at Granny's or have any break in routine. You want to give your child the best opportunity to establish and maintain what you will work on. Even if you keep up all the routines and strategies during a break away from home, sometimes this is not enough. You may find that all is well on your break, but it is a disaster when you return. For your and your child's sake, pick a three- to four-week period, batten down the hatches and focus on the task at hand. Thereafter a well-rested family unit can make all their necessary holiday plans and enjoy them!

Lucy Says

Set aside 3–4 weeks with no big changes.

Avoid sleepovers at Granny's and weekends away.

Don't implement your plan when vaccinations are due.

When to start

Working through sleep challenges can be a three- to four-week process – and that is provided that your child is well throughout. The first seven to ten days are generally the most challenging, but they are also the days when you will see the most improvements. You may even experience your first full night's sleep! Don't worry if you don't; proper sleep is imminent, provided you continue to implement the guidance and advice suggested. Don't waver; it will come. As the first week or so can be hard, it may be best for working families to begin the process going into the weekend. So start on a

Friday night and then 'own' Saturday and Sunday, when you have more control over your time. If you do shiftwork or irregular days, try to begin when you have a few non-work days in a row, or days off together before your child goes back to childcare, for example. You don't need to take a couple of weeks off work to help this happen, but the more provisions you can put in place to make the process easier for your family unit the better. For example, you might take Friday and Monday off and start on Thursday night. It won't be fixed within this time, but you should have covered significant ground.

Lucy Says

Starting on a Friday at bedtime can be a good idea for many families.

On the day you plan to start, get through the previous night as you normally would. Get up after 6 a.m. if your child is awake and alert, or wake your child no later than 7.30 a.m., even if you have to use your usual tactics.

Then you will follow the timetable that reflects your child's age as best as you can, but you will achieve sleep as you normally would – feed/rock/walk/buggy – with your main focus on getting your child plenty of sleep in anticipation of making the significant changes at bedtime. Then, from the second day onwards, you can address naps in the cot, if that is what you would like to achieve.

Lucy Says

On the day you start, operate the timetable provided but use your usual tactics to achieve the day sleep. Then make the suggested changes from dinnertime onwards. Start at bedtime with the new approach and operate it overnight. From day two onwards, begin naps in the crib with the new approach.

Get out and about

Being active and getting out and about is important for both parent and child. Fill your child's sensory diet with nature and fresh air. Exposure to bright natural light helps to improve sleeping patterns and all our children need this.

Lucy Says

Get some outdoor activity and fresh air; at least one hour per day. I recommend 30 minutes in the morning and 30 minutes in the afternoon.

As your child gets older you will really need to get up and out and encourage high-level activity during the day. Obviously, when you are tired from ongoing sleep issues, it can be hard to be motivated, but make it part of your plan. Your emotional and mental health will be enhanced.

Where do you want your child to sleep?

The choices are usually: in their own cot or bed in their own room; or in a cot or bed in your bedroom. If you want them to sleep in their own cot in their own room, we shall begin on that basis. Before any sleep learning exercise is implemented, I will always address the sleep foundations that are described in the next chapter.

However, some families are still not sure what to do, so I will help you make the decision.

It is generally advised that the child sleeps in the parents' room for at least the first six months of life, but many parents want to make the transition before the baby reaches this age. One option is to move the child into their own room before six months, but for one parent to share the child's room until they feel it's the right time to move back to their own. That way nothing will change for your child – they will remain in situ. Bear in mind that any change you will make can have an effect, so every decision needs to be treated with sensitivity.

Lucy Says

Decide where you want your child to sleep:

- Your bedroom
- Their own room
- In a bed with parent(s)
- In a cot
- In their own bed.

Currently room-sharing and/or bed-sharing

If your child is currently in your bedroom and maybe even in your bed, consider the following: If they were sleeping all night, where would they be sleeping? In their own room in their own cot or bed? Or in your bedroom but their own cot?

If you ideally want them in their own room but they currently are in _your_ room, then move them into their own room just before you begin the sleep learning process. Use my suggestions below to help ease them into this transition. If you are committed to them sleeping in their own space, then this is an important decision at the _start of the exercise._ Studies show that children sleep better in their own room, so if space allows – and it is age-appropriate and your preference – start preparing to move them out. It is fair to suggest that both the child and the parent can disturb each others' sleep.

If you are concerned about this move, have been practising a family bed approach or if your child is older than nine months, you can always room-share with *them* for the first three nights of the process to help bridge the gap. Even if you don't have a bed in their room or space for one, be creative; create a camp bed, just at the start. Many parents are very confident at this point and are happy to move the child into their own space with no transition period, but if you are in any way unsure, begin with the room-share swap and review after the first few nights. If your child has been breastfeeding, it may be best if dad does the room-sharing and mum is just available for whatever feeds are required.

Sibling room-sharing

One obstacle may be that you want siblings to room-share but you are afraid of them waking each other. For sibling-sharing to work I suggest that all parties need to be able to sleep through the night before being in a room together, and then you can set some ground rules about sharing and respecting each other's sleep.

If one child sleeps, but the other doesn't and that child is currently in your room as a result or you keep hooking them out of the shared room every time they wake and you are about to begin working on this, consider moving your *good sleeper* into your room or a spare room for a while and putting your current poor sleeper – *soon to be great sleeper* – on their own in the bedroom that they will eventually share. If you are afraid of upsetting or derailing the sleep of your other child, think carefully about this, but the main priority should be to avoid any changes for the poor sleeper once the issues are resolved. A second, less preferred option may be to move the child we are working with into a spare bedroom or for the parents to move out of their room just while you fix the problems.

If you are parent to multiples then I would generally keep them together unless you don't want them to share. Multiples have an unbelievable ability to sleep with each other and even if they don't initially, if you want them together then they need to learn to sleep with each other, so I would leave them together from the start.

However, have a good think about this and understand that you won't really want to make any fundamental changes to your child's sleep environment soon after correcting your issues, when you have worked so hard on making the improvements.

Planned room-sharing

If, on the other hand, you plan to room-share for an extended period of time, or space constraints dictate that parents and child must room-share, it is still possible to achieve great sleep. Of course it can be more challenging for the child, especially if you are planning on breaking a bed-sharing dynamic, but we do the best that we can in the circumstances. It can be a good idea to move the cot as far away from the parents' bed as possible. Very often this is not possible either, so it may be useful to swap sides of the bed with mum and dad, especially if mum has been breastfeeding.

The best time to move a child into their own room is between six months and eight and a half months of age; that way they have limited object permanence and their memory has not yet caught up. Any move after this age probably requires a few days of the room-share swap outlined above, where the parent room-shares for the first three days of the exercise and then goes back to their own room.

Bed sharing

If you are currently operating a bed-sharing dynamic some or all the time, you also need to decide if you want that to end. Common presentations are:

- Your child starts off in their cot and at some point in the night they come into your bed.
- They start off in your bed, get transferred to their cot and make it back into your bed at some stage overnight.
- They start off in your bed and stay there all night.
- Your child starts off either in your bed or their cot and you bring them into bed but not until a designated time, like 3 a.m. or 5 a.m., or out of sheer desperation.

If you are practising something along these lines and you want your child to sleep in their cot in their room all night; or you want them to sleep in their cot in your room; or you don't mind them coming into your bed early in the morning, you *will* need to make a clear decision. Unfortunately, most children who are recovering from a sleep problem will not be able to tolerate a bit of both arrangements – they need a consistent message. Some children successfully combine cot and bed-sharing and it suits everyone. But if you are trying to 'fix' your child's sleep and help them learn to stay asleep all night in their own defined place of sleep, you need to break the cycle of full or occasional or 5 a.m.-only bed-sharing from the start. In my experience, if you continue to bed-share from 5 a.m. onwards, for example, the waking time typically starts to get earlier and earlier until the waking turns back into nighttime activity with

'Is this the time?', 'Is it time yet?' wake-ups from your child until you eventually bring them into your bed.

Breaking the cycle of bed-sharing doesn't mean that you can't in the future enjoy Saturday morning pile-ins or cuddles in bed, but to avoid confusing your child, cutting this out at the start is the fairest approach. Don't forget, there is a large behavioural component to sleep. Intermittently reinforced behaviour is the most challenging to change and a significant barrier to sleep success, so please try not to operate an occasional tactic if you are committed to changing the current situation.

Planning to continue bed-sharing

If you plan to continue to bed-share with your child, you may find it takes longer to resolve the issues and night waking continues, but as you are in close proximity you will be able to successfully comfort your child back to sleep with minimised disturbance. You may well find weaning from the breast in this context very challenging, but once you are clear about what is appropriate for your family you can proceed with confidence. If you are committing to the family bed from bedtime onwards you will have to think very carefully about safety once your child is mobile. Many families will put the mattress on the floor and ensure that there are no areas of safety concern – open shelving, ability to wander out of the bedroom without parental supervision and so on. One option would be to work on bedtime in the cot and then bring the child into the family bed on first wake-up and commit to that sleeping arrangement, observing safe sleep at all times. For safe sleep guidelines for bed-sharing, see Chapter 4.

Cot versus bed

I normally recommend keeping toddlers in the cot for as long as possible and don't usually suggest making the transition to a bed until around two and a half to three years of age. At that stage your child has the reasoning ability to understand words like 'Stay in your bed all night.' You want your young child to have some impulse control and that when you issue an instruction they not only understand what you are saying but they can also make an effort to comply.

Often I see parents making the move to the big bed significantly sooner, usually in an effort to improve sleep, before this developmental skill set has emerged, and while many parents find that this early transition is seamless, others find that it only works because they are lying down and staying with their child at bedtime and also sleeping with them during the night, either in their bed or the family bed. This may not be desirable for your family unit in the long term.

If your young child is inclined to climb out of the cot and is at risk of injury, rather than trying a big bed before the recommended age range, try a learning exercise to teach your toddler necessary behaviour for the cot (such as 'no climbing') and supervise and encourage them while they learn.

Lucy Says

If your child is inclined to climb, don't necessarily react with introducing the big bed too soon; help them learn to stay in the cot without being a danger to themselves.

In a bed too soon

At least two or three times a week I meet parents in my practice with toddlers who are in a big bed too soon for their stage of development. These are typically children aged between 15 months and two and a half years who have ongoing sleep problems.

The parents often report: He doesn't like the cot; he is too big or too tall for the cot; she screams when put in the cot; he sleeps better in the bed; she will climb out of the cot.

Although all these concerns are valid, and we can discuss them in greater detail here, most of the time children under two and a half who are in a big bed and who don't sleep well have typically made the transition too soon. You may need to reconsider this if you hope to help your child become a better sleeper.

One of the largest contributory factors in ongoing sleep issues is parent dependency, at bedtime or during the night, or both, and if it is your intention to address this issue, one of the primary elements will be weakening the parent dependency at bedtime and overnight; and this is where difficulties may arise if the child is too young to be in the bed. Most children from 18 months onwards can begin to understand instructions such as 'Close the door', 'Put the rubbish in the bin', 'Pick up your toy'. However, what is absent until closer to two and a half years old and beyond is impulse control. This means that although the child can interpret instructions, they may lack the ability to see that command through – 'Stay in your bed', 'Don't get out when I leave the room', for example. So if a child under two and a half is in a bed you may struggle to keep your child in the bed when you are no longer present. One parent reported returning their 20-month-old to the big bed 137 times before finally giving up and staying beside him to keep him there, thus fuelling and not resolving his sleep issues.

Not all young children struggle in this way, and many families report that their youngsters sleep perfectly in toddler beds from 18 months onwards; and not all parents who *are* required to stay at bedtime need to repeat this exercise throughout the night. However, what we are discussing here are the problematic ones: those who are in a bed too soon, who require your presence at bedtime and/or who wake frequently throughout the night.

1. As we've seen, most young children are not ready to transition to a big bed until they are at least two and a half. If your child is sleeping well in the cot, there is no hurry – you can wait until they are three years plus. Resist the urge to make the change prematurely, even if a new baby is on the way. Often wonderful sleepers transform into horrible sleepers if this transition is rushed. Once your toddler is toilet trained or is close to it, this may be a good yardstick for comprehension

and impulse control. Applied in this time frame the transition can be seamless.

2. For those young children who appear to hate the cot and/ or always scream when put in the cot, parents must come to understand that this stems from a historic poor relationship with the sleeping space. All too often these children are not independent sleepers from infancy and they have been repeatedly transferred to the cot already asleep at bedtime, only to waken with a fright in the night to discover that their initial sleeping location has changed. The parental response is to immediately lift the child out of the cot and therefore perpetuate the cycle of insecurity. I encourage parents to help their children learn to feel safe and secure in the cot environment, initially with some acclimatisation exercises (detailed in the next chapter) during non-sleep time and then helping them start off their nighttime sleep in the cot when they are awake, using the stay-and-support approach. This way you can help bridge the gap between them hating the cot and learning to feel safe and content to sleep there.

3. Some young children may appear to sleep better in a bed because there are fewer changes once they go to sleep. Before they moved to the big bed, you may have transferred your child to the cot already asleep and they woke very frequently. When they moved to the big bed, you perhaps stopped changing the sleep location once asleep and this, in turn, minimised sleep interruptions, but did not resolve them entirely.

4. Many parents feel that their child is too big or too tall for the cot. They report that the child always bangs themselves on the bars and wakes themselves up. Typically, modern cots that meet current regulations are designed to accommodate even the tallest and biggest child. Kids that appear to thrash around the cot normally don't know how to *be* in the cot because they are put into the cot environment already asleep.

If your child began nighttime sleep in the cot from awake, this issue is typically resolved. If you are in any doubt about the size of your cot, purchase one that will eventually turn into a toddler bed, and that will remove any doubt about whether it is big enough.

5. Kids who climb. This is never a good reason to introduce the big bed prematurely. Obviously safety is paramount and you will need to ensure that your child cannot endanger themselves, but before panicking and making the transition too soon, teach your child not to climb in the cot. Most climbers realise that they can escape, but once the novelty has worn off, go back to sleeping in the cot without climbing. What you can do to prevent climbing is to ensure that they are getting lots of climbing and high-level activity time during non-sleep time. Teach them to go from standing to sitting to lying and make sure they understand the words that go with the actions. Put them into a sleeping sack to make it more difficult to get over the top of the cot – put it on backwards if necessary so they can't take it off. Supervise your child going to sleep and if they try to climb, gently push their knee down and explain 'no climbing'. Remove any items from the cot that help them to become taller – loose blankets, stuffed toys. Lower the setting to the lowest it can go, and lower again, manually if necessary – and safely, obviously. It may take time and patience but putting your child into a big bed should be the very last resort.

Once both parents agree that the safest, most appropriate place for their child to sleep is the cot, you can work on correcting and helping your child feel secure in the cot and reduce parental dependency at bedtime and overnight. The move to the big bed can wait and when you do make it, it should be seamless.

If your child is around two and a half years and in a bed, you will be interested in Chapter 6, which covers helping to package the plan for the older individual. If your child is younger and you are determined to keep the bed, by all means go ahead; but it may be more challenging than you anticipate and you may not achieve exactly what you set out to do.

Lucy Says

If your child is under two and a half years of age, it may be worth getting the cot back out while you work on the sleep issues. Your child could stay in a cot until three years plus. If you do decide to implement your plan with a bed, the process is the same. The only element that you may find challenging is when you start to move positions, you may find that your child will not stay in the bed without you being there and you will need to review and maybe adjust your sleep goals.

Keeping a sleep log

As you begin to implement the changes, start to keep a sleep log – a journal of what time your child woke, fed, napped, how long it took, bedtime, nighttime activity. Although this can feel like a chore, it is a worthwhile exercise to be able to analyse and review things on a daily basis. It will also help you to be objective about what improvements have been made week by week.

Chapter 3

Creating Positive
Supports For Sleep

A s you prepare to overhaul your current sleep practices, my priority is for families to lay a suitable foundation on which we can build a supportive sleep learning process. All the principles can be gradually introduced and each on its own can make a positive impact. Generally, however, most families find that they have to do everything in sequence – the positive supports; the age-relevant feeding and sleeping suggestions; and the sleep learning exercise – to get the best results.

Regardless of whether your child is already in their own room, in a cot or a bed or whether you are only now making adjustments, I suggest that you do some 'room work' to ease them into the process. This will later be reinforced by your bedtime routine and application of my supportive sleep learning approach.

Room acclimatisation

To begin with, start to spend lots of non-sleep time in the room. Use the room for activities other than sleep. I recommend that you allocate *at least* 30 minutes per day to room activities during non-sleep time. Change, dress and play with your child in their room, helping them to understand that it is a welcoming, safe place to be, and don't leave them alone. Many parents report that as soon as their child heads towards their bedroom they become agitated, stressed and upset, so these children need to be eased into liking their sleep space when it is not sleep time. Don't be worried that they will think that the room is for playtime – the environment or the stage that you set for sleep time will be somewhat different.

Cot exercises

Even if your child is used to going into the cot at sleep time and you feel that they are comfortable with the cot, it's a good idea to do some cot acclimatisation exercises. If your child is not used to going into the cot awake, or if they always cry when put down, or if they don't typically nap in the cot, or if they have never been in the cot that you bought before they were born, you should work on getting them to feel better about the cot as a safe environment.

Lucy Says

It is not unusual for young children with sleep issues to have a poor relationship with the cot, especially if you sneak them in there when they are already asleep and immediately lift them out into your arms or your bed when they wake. This can often create an insecure cycle where they feel unsafe and that is validated by you always taking them out when they cry.

Although these strategies are not a magic bullet, they go a long way towards changing the associations from negative to positive:

☑ Bring your child to the cot during non-nap/sleep times, every one or two hours throughout the day(s) before you begin the actual plan.

- [✓] Start by flying or circling baby in mid-air towards the cot and then lower them into the cot.

- [✓] Hold them firmly and safely, have their feet touch the mattress while you make a funny sound like 'bop', and reassure them verbally.

- [✓] Do this for maybe three to five minutes, gradually increasing the time their feet stay on the mattress.

- [✓] If your child is open to it, let them go, sit or lie your child down and play with them: maybe peek-a-boo with hands over eyes through the cot rails.

- [✓] Then pick the child up and leave the room.

- [✓] Over the course of the day, increase the time to five to ten minutes, see if you can hand your child a toy to play with or sit next to the cot and sing an interactive song like 'Itsy Bitsy Spider', or read a favourite book, then pick up and leave again.

- [✓] Repeat as frequently as you can, increasing the time and helping your child feel safe.

- [✓] Don't put them into the cot and go have a shower or put away laundry; put them in and stay and work with them

- [✓] This will help to teach your child to be calm in the cot and reassure them that you are not going to leave them.

- [✓] It can also help to teach *you* that your child won't necessarily scream or cry, and that they will become calmer.

- [✓] The primary goal is to interact with your child in the cot, the place where you want them to start to sleep, without any threat of you leaving and with limited or no tears. Once again, leave the room with the child and go off to do normal activities.

Acknowledging our children's senses can help them feel more calm and connected. Many of you instinctively leave your T-shirt or personal items (safely) with your baby to help them feel attached to you. Consider a similar approach where the cot is concerned, especially if you have been bed-sharing or using a sleeping place other than the cot.

Take the bedding from the cot, the sheet, the blankets, the sleeping bag and your child's sleeping clothes and sleep with them in your bed for a night or two. Then dress the cot in this gear on the night you begin. Your child will then smell their familiar sleep environment, the parent, that they associate with sleep and this can help ground their senses and instil calm.

The security item

I strongly recommend the introduction of a safe security item to use with your child for sleep. Many parents report that they have really tried using a security item but it has been rejected by the child. Very often the reason behind this is that the parent, or the bottle, or the dummy is the current security item and anything else is a poor substitute. If we begin to work on weakening those dependencies, the introduction of a lovey blanket or safe stuffed toy can start to take hold. Some children naturally have no interest, but I still encourage one at the start and if they are still not interested, fair enough. Others will begin to adopt the new item and it will stay with you for a long time. I have to confess that my own girls had no interest whatsoever in a security item but my boys very much embraced the concept for a very long time.

I am such a supporter of really trying to help this take as it can be so helpful for scary hospital stays, daycare and sleepovers, not to mention the fact that it is a great sleep cue – once handed the blanket in the cot, the child immediately assumes the sleeping position – so it is definitely worth pursuing.

When choosing an item be practical and consider at all times safe sleep. Due to the fact you can introduce a transitional item from very early on, ensure that it is safe and breathable and not too big. If necessary, discuss it with your GP. Whatever you pick, think whether you would panic if you saw it over your child's face; I suggest a piece of muslin, which is 100% breathable, about the size of a handkerchief so that it cannot be hazardous and, of course, it's easy to wash and have multiples of. Remember that, despite your efforts, most children will have a *grá* for a certain item!

At the start, sleep with the item and even consider wearing it inside your clothes. Include the lovey in your cot and room exercises – in peek-a-boo and other games – and also use it during your bedtime routine. Finally, tuck it in with your child at bedtime and nap times. Additionally, let your child have just *one* item at a time so that you do not create a prop scenario of *needing* one in each hand, for example, which can exacerbate the sleep problems that we are trying to resolve.

If you do all this and your child is just not interested, that may just be their personality type, like my daughters, or perhaps they have a dummy, and that is enough for them. At least you have tried.

Many experts instruct parents that you must only use the item at sleep time and, although I support the theory, I understand as a parent that sometimes kids like to bring their security blanket with them – you could meet me out and about with my youngest guy carrying his not very clean, well-worn lovey. That's a decision for you to make, but I don't see the harm. I know that my eldest son wouldn't be seen with his item once he started school, but it held a very special place in his room for many years after that.

Lucy Says

Select a safe, breathable and washable security item. A handkerchief size is good. Wear it and sleep with it first and then include it in the bedtime routine along with the cot and room exercises.

The dummy

You will always hear mixed reviews about using a dummy/soother/pacifier with young children. You may have promised yourself that you would never allow your baby to have one and yet you may find yourself using one after all. You may intend to use a dummy and find that your baby resists entirely. It is possible for your baby to seem uninterested in the dummy at first, only to become addicted to it; or you may find the reverse is true.

Using a soother in the early months of life can be a great way of helping to calm a fussy, unsettled baby. Sucking is hugely powerful in the first weeks and months of life and by using a dummy you can help to engage the calming reflex. It is possible to use the dummy between feeds, when your baby just wants to suck, not eat; provided that you have established your feeding routine. Furthermore, guidelines on Sudden Infant Death Syndrome (SIDS) suggest that using a dummy can help reduce the risk of cot death. Many reflux babies will also get relief from this sucking activity. Used like this, without dipping it in syrups or similar, and properly sterilised, a dummy can really help in the early days. However, you may need to think it through carefully. Although SIDS guidelines suggest that parents should continue using the dummy for the first 12 months (if it is used at all), always seek the advice of your GP before making any decisions. For more about SIDS and reducing the risk, see Chapter 4.

Lucy Says

Commonly, beyond four to five months of age, the dummy use can start to go against you. Suddenly, you may find that your baby wakes frequently and needs the soother to be re-plugged countless times overnight and during naps in the day. Indeed, your baby may only nap for 20–30 minutes and not return to sleep at all, or you may have to re-plug countless times to keep the nap going.

However, the dummy can become a sleep support that doesn't help. Parents should be mindful of the following: if your baby sucks to go to sleep, even if the dummy falls out of the mouth once asleep, most often the dummy will need to be replaced as your baby cycles through their natural sleep phases. It is a *sleep enabler*. This can mean that some parents replace the dummy 20 times or more during the night, involving considerable broken sleep for all. But don't worry if your baby has a dummy; in most cases you don't have to stop using it. In fact, well-rested children will need less and maybe no 'dummy runs' during the night.

Typically, countless dummy runs are caused by inadequate day sleep and bedtime being too late. A great night for a dummy-user is no dummy runs. A normal night would be one to three until you can teach your baby to use the dummy independently; this skill emerges around eight months, and even then you may still have to re-plug as they get stuck or fall out of the cot and the child needs help to find the soother. Excessive dummy re-plugs would be four or more during the night.

If you feel that having to get up and re-plug even two or three times a night is excessive, maybe you need to review your continued dummy use. Speak with your GP and decide what is appropriate for you. If your baby is six months plus and if you agree to discontinue the use of the soother, it is best dropped at bedtime as you begin to implement the other changes *and* the stay-and-support sleep learning approach that I will outline in Chapter 5. It is then advisable to discontinue using it throughout the night and into the following day for naps. It typically takes two to three days for a baby to get over the dummy and you can still use it for non-sleep time. If this is what you decide, it's nice to replace the dummy with a safe, breathable security item (see above).

Options with the dummy

If your baby is closer to eight or nine months it can become more challenging to take the dummy away and lots of parents see this as their only source of comfort and are reluctant to do so. This still doesn't mean that you should be getting up more than two or three times overnight. I suggest that you teach your baby to be independent of you in the context of their dummy and sleep. Always put the dummy into their hand and guide their hand to their mouth.

Over time, allow your baby find the dummy themselves by swiping their hand around the cot. I am not in favour of using more than one dummy at a time in the cot.

If you feel you want to offload the dummy at any age before 12 months and your GP agrees, go through the same procedure. It may be emotional at the start, but your baby will process the change within a few days.

If your child is still using a dummy beyond 12 months, you could be stuck with it until they are closer to two or even two and a half years of age, when you can explain your motives for taking away what may well be their security item by now.

If you are planning to stop using the dummy it can also be useful to start limiting daytime use for a few days in advance of the big night. If you attempt to drop the dummy and it is more stressful and emotional than you would like it to be, return the dummy and review the situation at a later date.

Once your child is two and a half to three years of age you may be able to bargain with them to discontinue the dummy. I would not suggest that you take this away and work on the sleep at the same time – it may be too stressful. Solve the sleep issues and review the dummy use at a later stage.

Lucy Says

Many families report that when they keep the dummy and once their child is 9 months or older, about one or two months after successfully achieving better sleep, the dummy runs disappear entirely.

Dummy retrieval

If your older child tries to keep getting you to come back to them or to return to the room by throwing their dummy out of the cot, I suggest you don't give that exercise too much air time or let it be a source of entertainment for your child. I recommend that you have a few spares in your pocket and when they throw the dummy, wait for three to five minutes and then give them one of the spares by slipping it into the cot and pointing to it, without verbal interaction. You can retrieve the original one at a later stage. Don't threaten your child that you won't give it back if they throw it – we both know you won't see that through – and also avoid using the dummy to get them to lie down or else you may become a performing seal. If you take the excitement out of this it will pass.

Dummy summary

☑ If your child is under eight months and has a dummy, they may struggle to find and replace it themselves. Remember – the more rested they are the fewer the dummy runs, but there may be more rather than less until they get older, and that is the nature of the dummy. But it will get easier once the skill emerges, at eight months plus.

☑ If your child is under nine months and you want to discontinue the use of the dummy, do so at bedtime, having made all the other changes outlined, and replace with my stay-and-support reassurance approach (see Chapter 5). Continue this approach overnight along with any other changes and into the following day. You can still use the dummy, if you like, for non-sleep times.

☑ If your child is between 9 and 12 months, you are likely stuck with the dummy until they are closer to two and a half years. Make the dummy work for you by always putting it into the hand and guiding the hand to the mouth. Over time, make sure that they make their hand look for the dummy and you will only have to get up a minimum number of times.

☑ Consider discontinuing the use of the dummy at around two and a half to three, but not at the same time as you address sleep – keep them separate. Sort out the sleep first and then the bargaining and bribing can begin.

Connected play and one-to-one time

As your sleep foundation is being laid, make sure that you are setting aside one-to-one time for both parents to spend with your child. Of course we spend lots of time with our young children, but very often this time is compromised with household chores, other family members, phones, television and electronic media. I know we are all guilty of checking emails or Facebook posts on our phone while we're having a conversation. One of the primary objectives when working on improving sleep is to ensure that you are emotionally available to your child both at sleep time *and* during the day. Twenty minutes of undiluted, exclusive time between child and parent can help solidify the bond, so make sure that you do this regularly:

- Allocate 20 minutes of exclusive time.
- Have face-to-face time instead of side-by-side time.
- Make sure that you have plenty of eye and physical contact.
- Get down on the floor with your child.
- Let them lead the play.
- Don't allow yourself to be distracted.

The sleep environment

I am always looking to establish positive associations with the sleep environment, wherever that is, and I would encourage you to implement some of the following suggestions.

1. Make sure that the room is sleep-inducing – in other words adequately dark. Blackout blinds and curtains are a great solution, especially for summer evenings and bright early mornings. It is also sensible to ensure that the room is dark enough for naps. It is important that you create the correct sleep environment for each sleep, not just for bedtime. Don't be concerned about your child confusing night with day; that phase has passed, and a dark room for day sleep is now of paramount importance.

2. Use a night light (4W) and avoid the use of external lights like hall lights, bathroom lights, ensuite lights, lamps on a dimmer switch, all of which can have a negative impact on your child's sleep. Actually, any other light, other than a night light, can stimulate the waking part of the brain before it should wake and it can also affect the retina at the back of the eye, interfering with the production of sleep hormones – even while your child is sleeping! I like the room to be dark but not pitch black. Your child should be able to see their hand in front of their face, find their dummy and see that they are okay, they started off here, they are safe and now they can roll over into their next phase of sleep. It's also useful to be able to manage your child overnight *without* turning on lights that will potentially arouse them more. If you or an older/other child are worried about the dark yourself, then use night lights in your hallway too.

3. Remove any distractions – cot toys, mobiles, mirrors, anything hanging from the ceiling, wardrobe doors left open, clothes hanging on the back of the door – anything that could over-stimulate or frighten your child. I have known mirrors to disturb sleep and I have witnessed a child chatting to the shadow of a towel. Lie on the floor in the dark in your child's room to view the room from their perspective. I suggest that the only thing that should be in your child's cot is their body, bedding and security item; anything else is a potential distraction.

4. Using a baby monitor in the room where your child will sleep may also help you as you work through the stages. Most families will invest in one in the early days and there are a number of options for parents, including sound, motion and video devices. Knowing that your child is safe and that you don't always need to disturb them to check on them may help you make a decision on whether you are ready to sleep separately from each other. Always position the monitor out of baby's reach. The night light feature can double up with

the night light that I recommend. If you find in time that the monitor is amplifying every move your child makes, once you are confident you can adjust the volume to suit.

5. Regulate the bedroom temperature and the clothes that your child wears. Your child will not sleep well if they are too hot or too cold, so dress them accordingly. The general temperature recommendation is 16–20°C, but make sure that you take your particular home into account. Ideally you want the temperature to be fairly constant with no big spikes or drops.

6. Consider the clothing for sleep. Dress your child appropriately for the season and your house temperature. I am a big advocate of the sleeping bag; it is a great sleep cue and can really take the hot and cold out of sleep as you can adjust it to the season. It can also help with a child who moves about a lot or kicks off blankets and, of course, it can help to immobilise a child who wants to stand and even attempt to climb out of the cot.

Lucy Says

Reconsider introducing the sleeping bag, even if your child has resisted this in the past.

Bedtime routine

Don't underestimate the power of the bedtime routine; a predictable sequence of events that happen in the same order, at around the same time and in the same place every night. It is that simple.

The premise of the bedtime routine is to bridge the gap between wakefulness and time for sleep and I suggest that you not only do this at bedtime, but for nap time as well. When you have an order of events at bedtime and follow the same procedure every night, it is a great sleep cue for your child – 'this is what happens to me when it is time for sleep'.

If the routine happens in the bedroom, where your child will sleep, this helps them to have positive associations with sleep and the room that they sleep in, which is very important. Sleep is a big separation and you want your child to feel safe and secure as they are drifting off. Spending 20–30 minutes of your time alone with them in their bedroom, relaxing them for sleep, will help to bridge this gap – and it can be an enjoyable time for both child and parent.

Lucy Says

Everything you do during your routine should be in a dim light, which will help to enhance production of the sleep hormone melatonin. Quiet, non-stimulating activity, with plenty of eye and physical contact, will help to regulate the heartbeat and increase production of the relaxing chemical oxytocin; and all these efforts together will help ease your young child into positive sleep.

Bedtime routines can start at any time from around six weeks of age, and it is never too late to start or to enhance an existing routine! I would advise that you avoid the use of television or electronics.

The perfect bedtime routine

1. Quiet the house an hour before bedtime. Turn off the television/computer. Spend one-to-one time with your child.

2. Finish any feeds in the living room or kitchen, so that you work towards weakening a potential feeding–sleeping association.

3. Consider a soothing bath to round off the day if you have the time. Alternatively, do a quick face wash and teeth brush and then go to your child's bedroom for the rest of the bedtime sequence.

4. Make sure that the bedtime routine happens in your child's bedroom to establish a really good connection between their room and sleep.

5. In the bedroom, dim the lights, pull the curtains and consider using white noise in the background, at the volume of a shower, to help regulate your child's heartbeat and relax them. Turn this off before they are asleep.

6. Consider some baby massage or some relaxing exercises for an older child.

7. Get your child ready for bed: change the nappy, put on the pyjamas and get them into their sleeping bag if you use one.

8. While getting your baby ready for bed, sing a particular song and say the same words over, so that they can learn the words that you say before lights out – 'Sleep time now, Harry, it's night night …'

9. Do some quiet reading or story-time with your child. Encourage them to look at the pictures and modulate your voice so that they are less inclined to want to eat the book. It's not the words that are important but the melodic way you say them. This quiet, non-stimulating time, with plenty of contact, can switch them from alert to sleepy.

10. If your child is book-adverse, get creative; do low-impact wooden puzzles, blocks, stacking cups, sorting shapes. What is important is that you are allocating this time in the bedroom, in the dim light, before sleep.

11. Provide a 20–30-minute wind-down. Build a process that you can add to as your child grows up.

12. Have an end to your routine; a certain phrase, turning off the lights or an 'I love you' ritual that signals the end of the routine and the start of your child needing to go off to sleep.

13. Then place your child in their cot – relaxed but awake – and use the stay-and-support approach (outlined in Chapter 5) if required.

Music, light shows and white noise

If you are going to use white noise or music it is important that it is used correctly. I generally recommend that you use it only during the bedtime routine and then turn it off. This also applies to light shows on the ceiling. The brain is very sensitive when going to sleep and can have a subliminal expectation that it should be on all night, which isn't always practical. The best option would be white noise over lullaby music, downloaded from the Internet – I like Harvey Karp – and set on repeat for the entire night. This will become a sleep association and as a result will need to travel with you. Your child can be weaned off it whenever you like, by just turning it down and eventually not turning it on. As with any change you make, it may take time for your child to acclimatise.

White noise can be very effective for young babies. You will also see later on in this book that I advise the use of white noise as distraction too. I would often suggest using white noise if you live in a busy apartment complex or have a noisy neighbour or dog, have an active toddler or are scared a new baby may wake your toddler. The white noise acts as a sound barrier and it should be on before sleep begins and should stay on for the duration of the sleep period. You can use it for all sleep periods or just for naps and not for nighttime, or vice versa.

Lucy Says

If you use white noise or music, it should ideally be turned off before your child goes to sleep, even if it turns itself off anyway within 15–20 minutes. Use only during the bedtime routine and then turn it off, unless you plan to use it all night long.

Chapter 4

Gentle Sleep-Shaping Approach: Birth to six months

It can be extremely challenging for some parents when your new arrival does not seem to 'sleep like a baby'. New babies *do* require an awful lot of sleep – some 12–16 hours per day – but this is rarely in large segments of time, and they have no respect for your nighttime sleep! *Their* sleep need is typically filled over a 24-hour cycle, feeding every 1–3 hours and sleeping every 1–2 hours for variable durations.

Childhood sleep is probably the biggest challenge faced by parents with an otherwise healthy child and it's not surprising that studies consistently support that 30–60 per cent of all families, depending on which study you read, have a potential sleep issue. As a new parent you may be alarmed to discover that sleep does not come naturally to your little baby and that they need considerable help from you in this department. Beautiful images of sleeping infants and well-rested new mums can be the opposite of the reality of becoming a parent and trying to get a handle on all your baby's requirements – feeding, winding, bathing, dressing and, of course, making sure that they (and you) are well rested. What comes naturally to some children, others may need extra assistance with; and that is *not* a reflection on you as a parent, it's more to do with your child's temperament and your journey. I often meet parents who tell me they think they have failed. I tell them immediately that that will not be the case. Sleep is challenging; there are many variations in what babies can do and it is not straightforward.

However, you *can* be proactive and work *towards* better sleep, without driving yourself crazy.

Lucy Says

Your new baby may need lots of assistance to achieve sleep and your task is to teach them to feel loved, safe and secure, not to be worried about 'bad habits'. Do what comes naturally.

Whatever your new baby's temperament – from easy to less easy – they all need a considerable amount of sleep within the first year, so don't be fooled into thinking that maybe *your* baby needs less than all the others just because they always seem to fight going off to sleep. Also, don't panic if your baby is not a 'good' sleeper; all babies can be programmed to sleep better in time.

Be prepared and realistic – *expect to be tired* as you embark on your new job in parenting, whether this is your first time or you already have children. It is a full-time, full-on position and every child is different. What works for some may not work for others. Just be fair to yourself and your baby; all sleep is a work in progress.

Lucy Says

While it is very normal for your new baby to sleep and feed little and often, it is also possible for parents to begin to lay a solid foundation for healthy sleep.

I really don't believe that a formal sleep learning exercise is appropriate for young infants especially not before six months and maybe even later, depending on the issues. That said, I am a firm believer in helping families to establish good sleep practices, if at all possible, in the early months – without putting anyone under any pressure. This is a very different time for your baby, with sleep biologically disorganised and their patterns mostly governed by the need to eat when hungry and sleep in between. That said, it is also a blank landscape within which you can start to put your imprint on better sleep, as soon as your child is able to. Here are some ideas about how to do this, but first, we will look at guidelines for safe sleep.

Safe sleep to reduce the risk of SIDS

☑ Always place your baby on their back to sleep.
  - Babies who sleep on their tummies have a higher risk of cot death.
  - It is not safe to place your child on their side.
  - When your baby is older and able to roll from back to front and back again, let them find their own sleep position, always having placed them on their back at the start of sleep.

☑ Keep your baby smoke-free before and after birth.
  - Smoking greatly increases the risk of cot death.
  - Don't allow anyone to smoke in the home or car.
  - If either parent smokes, you should not share a bed with your baby.

☑ Carefully think through bed-sharing based on the recommendations. Bed-sharing can also increase the risk of suffocation or entrapment. Do not share a bed with baby if:
  - either parent smokes (even if not in the home)
  - either parent has taken alcohol, drugs or medication, or
  - you are extremely tired.

OR

If your baby is:

- less than three months old
- was born prematurely (before 37 weeks), or
- had a low birth weight (less than 2.5kg or 5.5lbs).

☑ The safest place for baby to sleep is in a cot in your bedroom for at least 6 months.

- Place your baby with their feet to the foot of the cot so that they cannot get underneath the covers.
- Tuck covers in loosely and securely but not higher than baby's shoulders and ensure that they cannot slip over baby's head.
- Make sure your baby's head stays uncovered.
- Keep the cot free of loose and soft bedding, toys, bumpers, duvets, etc.
- Use a cot mattress that is clean, firm and flat and that fits the cot correctly. The mattress should be new for each child.

☑ Don't let baby get too hot.

- An overheated baby is at an increased risk of cot death.
- Don't wrap your baby in too many blankets.
- Cellular cotton blankets are best.
- Do not use duvets, quilts or pillows.
- Baby should not wear a hat.
- Ensure the room temperature is ranging from 16–20°C (62–68F).
- Never place the cot near a radiator, heater or fire, or in direct sunlight.

☑ Breastfeed your baby, if possible.

- Breastfeeding reduces the risk of cot death.
- Try to breastfeed for as long as you can.

☑ Consider a dummy.

- Some studies suggest that using a dummy each time your baby goes for a sleep reduces the risk of cot death.
- If you are using a dummy, then offer it at each sleep time.
- If you are breastfeeding, delay the introduction for a month until feeding is established.
- Don't worry if the dummy falls out when sleeping.
- Don't force the dummy if your baby is resistant.
- Don't attach the dummy with strings or cords.
- Never dip the dummy in sugar, syrup, honey or other food or drink.

☑ Provide tummy time with supervision. When your baby is awake, let them spend some time on their tummy and sitting up while you supervise.

- It is recommended to do this from birth.
- Always place baby on a firm, flat surface.
- Ideally, do this three times per day for 3–5 minutes and slowly build to longer sessions.

☑ Car seats, swings, infant seats and similar devices are not recommended for routine sleep in the house. Never fall asleep with your baby on the couch or armchair as the risk increases dramatically.

- Sleeping sitting up can cause problems with breathing.
- Once asleep, transfer your baby onto their back to sleep as soon as is practical.
- Babies should not be left unsupervised in a seated position for long periods of time.

If your baby seems unwell, get medical advice early and quickly. For more information, see sidsireland.ie.

A flexible feeding and sleeping rhythm

The early days and weeks should ideally be spent getting to know each other, learning about your new role and helping your baby learn to feel loved by providing for their every need. Although most parents don't want a strict routine, and I would agree, it can be very helpful if you do have some structure to your day and in turn your nights. A regular wake time between 7 a.m. and 7.30 a.m. is a good start. This will help anchor your first feed and regulate the body clock for daytime sleep. Bedtime will actually be quite late to begin with, but you *can* control the time you all wake to start the day.

Lucy Says

A regular wake time no later than 7.30 a.m. may be considered the first positive step to help ingrain positive sleeping practices from early on. Knowing what should happen next and when will give the new parent and the baby a sense of security and will also help you learn how to follow your baby's cues.

Without putting yourself under enormous pressure, follow the age-relevant suggestions in Chapter 9 to give you an idea of what you might aim for during the daytime. Some of this will occur naturally, some may not, but it can be a useful guide.

Learning to read your baby's sleep language

Getting to know each other is important. Interpreting your baby's sleep cues is extra important. Having a regular daytime structure can enable new parents to correctly read the baby's cues for both food and sleep and everything in between. Understanding what your baby might do when *starting* to get tired can also be the next positive step in appropriate sleep hygiene.

Early 'tired' signals – the ones that you need to acknowledge and act on – are:

- ☑ A brief yawn
- ☑ Momentary zoning out/staring/snuggling in

☑ Decreased activity

☑ A brief eye rub.

These signs indicate sleep readiness and, given the opportunity, most babies will be able to go to sleep with relative ease.

Late sleep signals may be represented by:

☑ Intense eye rubbing

☑ Wide yawning

☑ Increased activity – clenching fists/arching back

☑ Agitation

☑ Noise – whingeing/moaning/crying.

Any or all of the above indicates that your baby has become overtired. This may mean that they will struggle to go to sleep, even though they are super tired. You have missed their optimum time for sleep and now you may experience a struggle to get your baby to go to sleep, and sleep may also be of a short duration. This can make it very difficult to have a rhythm to your day, despite your best efforts. Getting the timing right for the onset of sleep can eliminate tension at sleep time and also promote longer sleep duration, both during the day and overnight.

Soothing strategies

A large percentage of babies are unsettled. Many find it difficult to sleep without some low to medium to high levels of parental intervention. We know that the skills to be independent of parents, in the context of sleep, may not emerge until six months plus, and even at that age may not emerge naturally, but need to be enhanced and improved by you.

Try not to worry about what you may perceive as 'bad habits' – there is no such thing in the early days. Don't take much notice of well-meaning advice that you are 'making a rod for your own back' or that your baby is 'playing you'. There is so much going on from a feeding and development perspective that if your baby needs a high level of support from you, then you must give it and do so guilt-free, knowing that it may diminish naturally, or you will be able to weaken it as they get older and they are more open to learning.

If this sounds familiar, rather than worrying, concentrate on developing coping mechanisms if your baby is unsettled. If your baby is struggling – wants to be up and on you, which is very typical – develop lots of ways of helping them to settle, other than just feeding. Teach them to respond to a variety of calming measures.

Lucy Says

Many young babies arrive requiring lots of support from you – they want to be rocked, held and comforted – and you should allow for this. It will pass in time.

Support your baby's needs with lots of holding – try different positions. Babies are big fans of motion – encourage rocking in your arms, or (safely) in swings and seats. Try not to get stuck with only one way of soothing baby – the more ways you can calm your baby, the easier it will be to phase out motion and unconventional sleeping places as your baby gets older.

Don't be afraid of using a dummy in the early days, especially if sucking helps to calm them. There's more on dummies in Chapter 3.

- Only introduce when feeding is established.
- Avoid dipping into sweet syrup or teething gel or medication.
- Ensure that the dummy is always sterile.
- Avoid using straps or string to secure the dummy.
- Don't worry! This doesn't have to be a long-term commitment.

Some motion suggestions that baby may respond well to:

- Baby slings and carriers
- Infant swings
- Pram/buggy
- Rocking in a rocking chair

- Car journey
- Vibrating seats
- Bouncing on exercise ball.

Lucy Says

Avoid leaving your baby in swings, car seats and bouncer chairs any longer than the manufacturer's recommendations.

Where will baby sleep?

Ultimately most babies will sleep in a conventional cot, but generally not until they are six months plus, as a cot may be too big a space at the beginning.

For nighttime and even some daytime sleep, the best options are probably a Moses basket or a crib that can be placed next to or attached to your bed (this is called a co-sleeper or sidecar). This sleeping space is normally temporary as your baby will get big quickly and then will perhaps move to a conventional cot. There are plenty of choices on the market and there are even some that transition from a newborn sleeping space all the way through to a toddler bed. Don't be overwhelmed; your decision will be based on your budget and your space and, of course, your preferences and parenting style.

It is likely that your baby will room-share with you for at least the first six months. Then, based on rooms available and on your own feelings about where you want your child to sleep, they may move out into their own bedroom.

- Your baby will benefit from a small space to feel safe at the start.
- Young children sleep better and longer in close proximity to their mums.
- You will *always* need to invest in a new mattress for each new baby. So keep this in mind if you are being given or lent a

Moses basket, crib or cot by family or friends. The mattress needs to be firm, meeting health regulations, and you should always place your baby into the crib with their feet close to the end.

- During the day and evening, you will probably want your baby quite close to you. At the start, they can have a tendency to sleep whenever and wherever with noise and light not really bothering them.

- The pram component to your buggy can serve very well as a crib. Your baby can lie flat and be comfortable and you can always roll them in the house, if you are not planning on a walk, to help them drift off to sleep.

- To begin with, your baby will have a late bedtime, so you will probably keep them with you in the living area in the pram, your arms or the Moses basket. When it is bedtime, you will all go to bed and the baby will be in the crib or Moses basket for the night (at least in theory).

- Although you may not plan to share your bed with your baby, planned and unplanned bed-sharing happens and there is nothing wrong with it. You shouldn't feel guilty about this approach to sleeping; in fact, it can help many mums get more sleep. Although the current health agenda does not support it, it would seem that as many as 70 per cent of parents share the bed at some stage. So if you are bed-sharing, whether planned or otherwise, ensure that you are observing safe sleep and providing a risk-free environment. Even if you *do* share the bed, it doesn't mean you can never reverse this situation. Consider returning your baby to the cot once they are 12–16 weeks plus to diminish their expectations of sharing the bed with you.

Quality sleep in the family bed

There is no one correct way to approach healthy sleep for your family unit. There are many different parenting styles and essentially it is a personal choice. Infant sleep can be hotly debated and, indeed, controversial. Decisions about where your baby will and should sleep are deeply personal and very often your views may change depending on your particular child.

Co-sleeping – also referred to as the family bed or bed-sharing – can be a great, connected approach for many families and it can work exceptionally well. However, many parents may find that although they have no issue with bed-sharing or co-sleeping with their children, nobody's getting any sleep. That still doesn't mean you have to give up sharing the bed, it may just mean you need to review the situation and make some adjustments to help the things work a little bit better.

First, as with any sleep approach, you need to observe safe sleep. Adult beds were not designed with safe infant sleep in mind, so the parents must ensure that the environment is risk free. Infants should sleep on their backs, on a firm, clean surface under breathable, comfortable bedding. Parents should remove loose bedding, stuffed toys and pillows and ensure that the infant is not too hot or too cold. Avoid using a hat for your sleeping baby. It is imperative that there are no gaps or spaces that put your baby at risk of getting trapped or suffocated. The environment should be smoke free. One of the most prevalent risk factors in SIDS is linked to smoking.

Never risk falling asleep with your baby on a sofa or armchair. If you're feeling really tired and think you may fall asleep with your baby while feeding or cuddling them on a sofa or armchair, move to a bed – bearing in mind the safety guidelines – or, if possible, ask your partner, a friend or family member to look after them while you get some rest.

When starting to bed-share all parties should ideally be committed and informed. Everyone sharing the bed should agree and be comfortable with this family-orientated decision and also acknowledge that everyone who occupies the bed is responsible for the safety and well-being of the child. Obviously, use of alcohol, drugs or medication is not recommended and those unable to wake easily should not co-sleep with the infant.

SIDS guidelines suggest that parents delay co-sleeping for the first three months, or if your baby was born before 37 weeks or had a birth weight under 2.5 kg/5.5 lb. However, many parents will co-sleep much sooner, especially when breastfeeding, as this is the most natural environment. Personally, I committed to this practice with my full-term (11 days over!) 8.6lb bundle of joy and it meant that we all got lots of sleep. Speak with your GP or health visitor if in doubt. The use of a 'sidecar' or 'co-sleeper' attached to the main bed can often be a very good alternative in the first instance. If you are bottle feeding it is advised that the baby sleeps on a separate surface alongside the mother rather than in the bed, so the 'sidecar' is the solution here.

Lucy Says

Carefully think through your co-sleeping environment as your baby gets older and increasingly mobile. Some families find that a mattress on the floor is a great solution once the baby is rolling and more agile. Once your child is on the move, consider room safety – install wardrobe door locks, remove bookshelves to prevent climbing and maybe even put in a stair gate to stop your child wandering unsupervised out into the hallway and close to the stairs.

Remember, there is no *right way* for sleep. It has to be what is right *for you* and it must be safe and risk-free. Whatever you decide, it can be adjusted and refined so that it is also sleep-enhancing for all involved. Parents should do what feels right for these first few months and then you can look at things again when your baby is older and more open to being separate from you – if this is what you want.

Lucy Says

Don't let yourself feel pressurised by popular theories about what is right or wrong. Find a sleeping space solution that works for you and your baby, even if it is not as you initially envisaged. Sometimes we have to make adjustments to our ideals depending on the child's temperament and needs.

A sleep-friendly environment

Although sleeping through the night won't come for quite some time and every baby is different, from early on, try to make nighttime sleep-friendly. Always take your baby up to bed at their bedtime, even if it's late at the beginning. Make sure that the room is sleep-inducing, with black-out blinds or curtains. Provide your bedtime feed and pre-sleep ritual in a dim light. Turn off the light when it is sleep time and avoid hall lights and bathroom lights; use only a 4W night light in the room or use the light from the baby monitor. Do nighttime feeds in the dark (use the night light if it is bright enough, or low lamplight) and keep the feed non-stimulating. Many experts suggest that you avoid speaking to or looking at your baby, but I don't advocate that approach. Enjoy nighttime parenting but don't over-stimulate. Be practical – the night feed should be brief, and the sooner everyone gets back to sleep the better. Keep the night feeds in the bedroom exclusively – changing the location may in time create an expectation and may wake your baby up fully. Once you are confident, change the nappy overnight only when you feel necessary and if it is, do so mid-feed, so that they can get sleepy in the second part of the feed.

Overheating

According to the HSE's safe sleep guidelines, overheating can increase your baby's risk of cot death. A baby can overheat when asleep because of too much bedding or clothes or because the room is too hot.

☑ To check how warm your baby is, feel their tummy – it should feel warm but not hot.

☑ If their tummy feels hot or if they are sweating anywhere, they are too warm, so remove some of the bedding.

☑ Other signs include flushed, red cheeks and fast breathing. Don't worry if your baby's hands and feet feel cool; this is normal.

☑ Avoid overdressing your baby – a nappy, vest and babygrow are enough. They can wear less in warm weather. Remember to take off baby's hat and extra clothes as soon as you are indoors.

☑ Make sure the room your baby sleeps in is not too warm. The room temperature should be 16–20°C. If the room feels too warm for you it is too warm for your baby. Consider buying a room thermometer.

☑ Never place the cot, pram or bed next to a radiator, heater or fire or in direct sunshine.

☑ Do not use too many blankets – sheets and light blankets or cellular blankets are best as you can adjust the temperature by adding a blanket or taking one away. Cellular blankets have small holes in them so they can keep your baby warm without overheating.

☑ Do not use duvets, quilts or pillows.

Establishing a bedtime routine

From as early as six to eight weeks of age your baby will begin to smile back at you. This means they are responding to social cues and so it is a perfect time to begin having a pre-sleep ritual, one that helps them to understand that what happens next is sleep time. It also helps wind your baby down in advance of sleep and take them from alert to sleepy. Once established you can then use this ritual before nap time as well.

Sample bedtime ritual

1. Dim lights

2. Change nappy/dress for sleep

3. Sing a series of songs

4. Use a certain mantra, e.g. 'Sleep time, baby'

5. Provide the bedtime feed

6. Place the baby in their sleeping space.

The percentage of wakefulness approach

This approach helps develop a sleep ability. Put your baby in the cot, more awake than asleep, specifically at bedtime, in order to encourage the ability to rely less on parents during the 'going to sleep' process. Sleep problems may start to emerge when your child is six months and older if they have not developed the ability to go to sleep without parental input. At this early stage you have the perfect opportunity to avoid ever having a sleep problem that is based on dependency.

Some babies come with a high need of support from you to get through the day. However, they also come designed to be able to start doing some of the hard work at sleep time, but only if you give them space and opportunity. You need to be patient, allowing them to be partially, if not wholly, independent of you at sleep time as they get older.

Bedtime, albeit late, is the best time to practise and enhance this skill set initially. Try to avoid always having your baby completely asleep at bedtime and encourage them to do some of the work of falling asleep themselves. This can be the next positive step to ensuring that you avoid long-term sleep difficulties.

Initially your baby will potentially be 100% asleep before you put them into their sleep space at bedtime.

Once you have begun getting a sense of regularity to the day and you are observing your baby's sleep language and have developed a bedtime routine, the next step is to try to have them less than completely asleep at bedtime. I refer to this as the percentage of wakefulness because most of us can envisage what 100 per cent asleep looks like and in turn can envisage what 95 per cent asleep and 5 per cent awake might also look like!

Get your baby to the point of sleepiness and start putting them into the cot *before they are entirely asleep*. If they fuss and squirm and moan a bit, gently reassure them with physical support such as rubbing, stroking and tapping them, and verbally support with shushing or gentle singing. If your baby is increasingly upset, pick up and comfort back to sleep and try again in another day or so. If you keep working through this procedure, gradually – and specifically at bedtime – they will become more *aware* of being put down and actively finding a sleep state with less involvement from you. As a result, you are laying a path to a sleep ability that will work in your favour as time goes by.

The idea is that you work through the process, but you don't continue if your baby is not tolerant and cries terribly for comfort and support. This would indicate that they are not ready and to persevere may be unfair – never try to get better sleep at the child's expense. However, keep trying it and if they never seem ready, you can continue with *all the other sleep recommendations* and move it up a gear as they head to six months onwards with my stay-and-support approach, outlined in Chapter 5.

Lucy Says

Don't worry if at first your baby does not respond well. Try again at a later stage.

Dummy tip

If you are using a dummy, you can try to weaken the association of dummy with sleep, consequently reducing the need to re-plug countless times, by practising removing it before your baby is entirely asleep in their sleep space. If your baby roots for the dummy, push up the chin when they are rooting; if they become upset, return the dummy and repeat as many times as required until your child goes to sleep without it. Once again, you may need to judge the effectiveness of this approach as it can sometimes be an exercise in frustration for all! See my thoughts on long-term dummy use in Chapter 3.

Some gentle natural solutions

☑ In the first four to six weeks, teach your baby the difference between day and night by using exposure to light during the day and waking times and using dim lights for nighttime. This will help regulate the body clock and start to lay a foundation for healthy and lengthier sleep. Beyond 10–12 weeks of age parents may start to see a daytime structure appear and can look forward to longer stretches overnight.

As baby gets older the need to distinguish between day and night becomes less relevant and I encourage a dark environment for all sleeps thereafter as the body naturally makes this distinction.

☑ Get plenty of fresh air and outdoor activity. Studies support that young infants who get outside, specifically in the afternoon, sleep better and longer than those who do not. There is a suggestion that babies are more active in the light, and light influences the early development of the biological clock. This regulates many body functions, such as the secretion of the sleep hormone melatonin which plays a key role in well-balanced sleeping patterns.

☑ Ensure adequate daytime sleep as per the sleep suggestions provided. Do your best to make sure that your infant is well rested throughout the day. Don't worry if your baby will only sleep on the go or in arms – in the short term this is a good strategy – the more rested they are, the better they will sleep at night. Parents can work on phasing out motion sleep when they are older and more open to learning.

☑ Keep your baby close to you. Room-sharing is recommended anyway for the first six months, but as well as the benefits of reduced risk of SIDS, studies also indicate that sleeping within close proximity to mum can regulate the baby's sleeping patterns. Night feeds can be done with minimum disruption, too.

☑ Use white noise. The sound that mimics the womb/heartbeat or the noise of a radio, extractor fan or hair dryer can have an instant calming effect on baby. Don't use the actual appliances (for safety reasons); you can download apps or purchase CDs. Don't use white noise turned up too loud for an extended period of time and move the device far away from your baby's ear. Don't underestimate its immediate power to distract and then regulate the heartbeat, increase the alpha waves in the brain and actually help the baby fall asleep faster and deeper. If your baby goes to sleep listening to white noise, it should stay on for the entire sleep period.

Don't worry about needing it long term; you can wean the baby off it by gradually turning it down.

☑ Use a baby monitor for peace of mind when you are not with your baby. Decide on the one that suits your family best and then ensure that it is positioned at least one metre away from the baby.

☑ Learn infant massage. Babies who have been massaged before sleep time fall asleep more easily and into a deeper sleep. Along with the sleep benefits massage can also improve digestion, growth and development as well as providing a perfect bonding opportunity.

☑ Make sure that you are continually encouraging tummy time from six weeks onwards throughout the course of the day, even if your baby doesn't seem to like it! Commit to 5 to 10 minutes every waking hour. Get creative and use the floor or the bed (with supervision) and get your baby rolling. By four months I really do like to see this skill emerge and it will help your child sleep; they will be able to get comfortable and sleep in a natural position.

Reflux and intolerances

One of the most stressful difficulties for parents of a young infant can be reflux and milk intolerances.

A baby with reflux can be much more than a laundry problem. It can be a living nightmare for many parents, with cases ranging from mild to extreme. As many as 1 in 10 babies are diagnosed within the first few months, though many outgrow it within 6 to 12 months. It can be difficult to experience the pain and discomfort that a baby suffering with this condition may feel, leaving parents frustrated and drained as they try to seek answers from a variety of sources. If you are concerned that your baby may be suffering from this condition, please seek advice from a medical professional. A lot of cases can be managed by a combination of medication and interventions from a wide circle of sources, such as changes in formula, adjusting the breastfeeding mother's diet, cranial osteopathy and sacral therapy and feeding and sleeping positions.

To make things even more stressful, reflux and intolerances can have a significant impact on your baby's sleep. Once these problems are controlled, there's generally no reason why your baby can't go on to be a great sleeper; it just may take extra time as you discover the extent of your baby's issues and you may be left with unhelpful sleeping associations because of the reflux. Some reflux babies also have food sensitivities and food intolerances, which can further wreak havoc on healthy sleep; common symptoms, outside pain and discomfort, may be really frequent nighttime awakening, restless sleep and/or long wakeful periods overnight. You will need to work closely with your paediatrician, GP and health visitor. Until the issues are treated and adequately under control it may be impossible to expect your baby to sleep through the night or for any length of time. In the meantime, you can try to create a framework so that better sleep will soon follow and that you survive the rollercoaster of reflux.

1. Use the age-relevant feeding and sleeping suggestions. Don't ignore the advice about waking no later than 7.30 a.m. so that you regulate the body clock and align your feeding plan for the day. A baby with reflux may benefit from feeding little and often, but make sure that you anchor the day with your first feed within 30 minutes of waking to avoid sleeping and feeding clashing throughout the day. Feeding little and often can sometimes make the situation worse. Although it appears to help your baby cope, it can also mean that they never take a full feed and therefore you never manage to get into an age-appropriate daytime schedule. It would be preferable to get the symptoms under control and then have your feeds and sleeps properly paced and balanced throughout the day. If you are providing medication, do this immediately on waking so as not to delay the first feed any further.

Lucy Says

Throughout the day try to get into the habit of
feeding on wake-up to avoid the overlay of feeding
and holding that may start to become a sleep
dependency as time goes by.

---

2. With a regular timetable you can then help to plan when sleep should happen. Reflux babies may be harder to read than other young infants. Early sleep cues may not be that apparent and you may do better focusing on the time on the clock. Watch out for the early signs of getting tired – brief eye rub, yawn, zoning out. The wakeful period first thing can be really quite short, with some babies under six months requiring a nap within 45 minutes of waking up – this is obviously made more difficult if you have to hold the baby upright for 20–30 minutes post-feed. Allowing overtiredness to ensue first thing in the morning can mean you have to firefight all day with an overtired *and* refluxing baby. I would suggest that you try to prepare for a nap within a maximum of an hour and forty minutes from wake-up in most babies up to eight months. It may be helpful to keep a sleep log, which may help identify the right times for sleep. When you do think that it is time for sleep, bring your baby to a quiet/ dark environment to help them unwind and in turn their sleep signs may become more apparent.

3. Discuss sleeping positions with your GP or health visitor. Babies who are uncomfortable may not settle well on their backs, despite the SIDS awareness agenda supporting 'back to sleep'. Try having your baby sleep on their left side once they are old enough to do so. Look into a wedge or other support products, which can help. ClevaMama® has a great range of suitable sleep positioners and supports.

4. Practise lots of tummy time, despite any protestation. Do this little and often; it will help develop your baby's ability to roll onto their tummy and back again, which in turn allows them to get into a comfortable position for sleep. This promotes the ability to get comfortable without parental input.

5. Elevate the cot. You may also need to create a little nest at your baby's feet to stop them slipping down; and, of course, at all times observe safe sleep.

6. If your baby is very irritable and things are very difficult, don't worry about where daytime sleep happens, just try to make sure that it does happen – buggies, cars, slings, swings can all help your baby get well rested even when they are not 100 per cent comfortable. Concentrate initially on the bedtime percentage of wakefulness approach. Later, when the medical conditions are managed, you can focus on more conventional sleep-friendly, stationary day sleep environment and, of course, the overnight, when your baby is more robust and feeling more comfortable.

7. Make sure that you dress your baby comfortably for sleep. Try to use outfits and sleepwear that are loose at the waist.

Lucy Says

As with all parenting difficulties, this time will pass. Seek support and advice from family, friends and your healthcare providers to help you survive this time and so that you and baby ultimately thrive.

Signs and symptoms of reflux:

☑ Frequent vomiting, both through the mouth and sometimes through the nose. Be mindful that not all children actively vomit; some have silent reflux, which means that the acid comes up, causing pain, but there is no vomiting.

☑ Some reflux babies, but not all, may be slow to gain weight.

☑ Reluctance to eat, or at least stay on the job. Initially keen and then arching away from the breast or the bottle, causing the feeds to be disturbed, or wanting food little and often.

☑ Constant hiccups, choking or gagging.

☑ Sour breath.

☑ Chronic irritability, excessive crying for long periods of time in the day.

☑ Discomfort when lying on their back.

☑ Sleep disturbances, waking frequently, often seemingly in pain.

☑ Chronic cough/congestion.

See your GP or healthcare provider to help you get to the bottom of these issues. Once managed you will be able to build towards better sleep.

Chapter 5

Stay-and-Support Sleep Learning Approach: Six months to two and a half years

If your child has an over-reliance on parental presence – a feed or nurse or to be held, for example – to achieve and maintain their sleep, the introduction of positive supports may need to be augmented with a sleep learning exercise. You may be aware of techniques that are referred to as 'shush, pat', or 'pick up, put down' or, of course, 'cry it out'. These are all strategies used to break a cycle of parental dependency. Through many years of working with families I have devised an effective, considerate, attended approach modified from the various sleep settling techniques, that allows parents to stay and support their child as they learn a new way of going to sleep and then gradually scale themselves out of the room.

Don't apply this strategy without following the feeding and sleeping suggestions outlined in Chapter 8 as the two elements require each other in order to be 100% effective.

For parents this may be the unpleasant part of the process – no one sets out to have a sleep problem and very few parents like their child to cry and be upset. I cannot provide assurances that my strategies allow for no crying, but I can say that everything we are doing here is designed to minimise crying and upset and that generally the crying is short-lived and, more important, entirely parent-attended. It is not possible for me to tell you exactly how your child will respond – these factors are influenced by your child's temperament, age, what you have been doing, what you have tried in the past, what message you have given your child and how long the issues have been going on.

There is not really an ideal age for this process: I work with children up to six years and each age bracket comes with its own challenges. Some children are a dream to work with; others will put you through your paces. Although that can be hard, what is important is that once you begin, you see it through, and that you understand that this is *your child's journey*; you need to be patient and committed and focus on one step at a time. Avoid worrying about the 'what ifs' – 'what happens when we ...?' As my grandmother would say, don't meet trouble halfway. Let's take it a few days at a time, otherwise you will be overwhelmed by the entire process and your fear and anxieties can be a barrier to success.

Lucy Says

Try not to be overwhelmed. Take each part of the process in small increments and you will start to see improvements – in mood, behaviour, appetite and sleep! Most parents report that the process was not nearly as hard as they imagined and that each day they felt more confident and capable and indeed proud of their child as they developed a new skill set.

I suggest that although you *may* be challenged in the short term, it is all for long-term gain and an improvement that will have a positive knock-on effect in every part of your parenting. High-need babies become more easy and relaxed; children and parents can be happier; and parents have the opportunity to recapture a part of their life before children, which is also important. Time together in the evening and both parents sleeping in the same bed can often be a bonus or a rarity if you have a child who does not sleep.

Ultimately the decision is yours to make as a family. Often just introducing the positive supports and aligning them with the age-appropriate timings in Chapter 8 are enough for some, but if you want to weaken the dependencies and help to further create a happy solo sleeper, here is the brief for you to work from.

Who should start?

If both parents are available and either can put your child to sleep at bedtime using your usual tactics, I would describe your child as interchangeable and then it doesn't matter who starts. Sometimes dad may feel that he will be stronger and mum feels that she will be stressed about crying, and sometimes the reverse is true. In this instance, just have one parent operating at bedtime on nights one and two and the second parent to provide the new approach on nights three and four and then alternate.

It's best if both parents are involved. If just one parent is always 'fixing' things, there are no learning opportunities for either parent. So alternate whenever possible, even if long working hours mean that one parent is around less than the other. When possible both parents should become efficient at this new sleep practice.

If your child responds better generally to mum, for example, mum should start; but dad should definitely get involved before too long, if at all possible.

If your child is breastfed or has been breastfed until recently, the other parent most certainly should operate on nights one and two and then the breastfeeding mum on nights three and four, and then they should alternate thereafter. In this instance the other parent may feel that baby just would not respond and that whenever they have tried in the past the child has gone berserk ... but give it a try. Mum must agree to give both parties a chance and not rescue baby, in an effort to build a trusting sleep relationship between the two. If baby is really not settling, I would reintroduce mum but also let dad keep trying. If this is still ineffective, I get the responsive parent to take over for seven days and then try again.

If you are parenting solo, I suggest that you draft in support – a sister, friend or parent – if possible, not necessarily to implement the plan, but to be there for you emotionally in the first few days.

If you have other children, you will need to ensure that both parents are around in the evening to supervise the other children, or engage a babysitter or someone to help you so that you do not leave a child unsupervised and feel uncomfortable about this as well, especially as you start. I know that the budget doesn't always extend to this, but it will only be at the start.

Many families are parenting alone, or dad is away working, and if you need to be supported, call on your friends. After a few days, you won't need them, but they can help at the beginning.

How to begin

- ☑ You will follow the feeding and sleeping suggestions for your child's age group outlined later in the book.
- ☑ You will have offered the bedtime feed at least 45 minutes before bedtime, well separated from sleep.
- ☑ You will provide a calm, consistent bedtime routine.
- ☑ You will turn off the lights and white noise/music.
- ☑ You will gently place your child into the cot awake and relaxed or have them climb into their bed.

Position yourself beside the cot or bed and start using the stay-and-support settling techniques outlined.

For parents who don't normally stay with their child at bedtime and feel that they are already independent at this stage of the bedtime process: walk away as you normally do, provided they are calm. If they are not calm (this can happen – while some of the changes are subtle, they can cause your usually calm bedtime process to unravel), return to the room, position yourself beside the cot and start to use the stay-and-support approach brief outlined below.

Lucy Says

If you don't normally stay at bedtime and your child
falls asleep really quickly when you leave, you may
find that these changes unhinge that process and your
child struggles to go to sleep as easily. Don't panic –
this is already progress. Return to the room and go
through the process outlined below. Understand that
the ease with which your child was going to sleep
initially was possibly part of the problem.

The stay-and-support approach

This approach can be used at bedtime, overnight and for naps.

When you have completed your bedtime routine, position
yourself on the floor (or a chair, but only if your child's cot is
still at the high level). Get down to your child's level, low on the
floor beside the cot or bed, where you can easily comfort, reassure,
support and emotionally engage with your child as they learn the
process of sleep.

Lucy Says

Be low on the floor unless your child's cot is still at the
high level.

Make yourself comfortable – it may take some time!

Be patient and calm; it takes time to learn something new. This is
progressive learning on your child's part.

Physically respond to your child

You can comfort your child physically by stroking, rubbing and
patting through and over the bars of the cot or from beside the bed.
Touching your child will let them know that you are there and help

to regulate their autonomic nervous system. Consider what your child likes.

You could:

- Stroke the temples
- Stroke the bridge of the nose
- Rub the back of the neck
- Do a pat, pat shush on their side or torso
- Walk your fingers up their body
- Swirl your hands over their tummy
- Do a tom-tom rhythm on their body
- Roll them on their side
- Wiggle their torso.

You should do this intermittently, trying to avoid creating a new sleep association, but at the same time being aware of where you are coming from. You can ease off on this as the days go by, but it is a great 'in-between' for parents.

Try to ensure that you, the parent, are in charge of the touching. Avoid allowing your child to fall asleep holding your hand or finger. If they grab you, pat or rub a different part of the body, tuck their hand in with their security item. If you *remain* hand-holding at sleep time you may wake your child as you try to leave and ingrain a hyper-vigilance around falling asleep. You may also have to start the settling techniques all over again.

Lucy Says

If you are weakening hand-holding as your sleep issue, try to stop completely from night one onwards or use a security item between your hand and theirs. Concentrating on a different part of their body will help them transition, and you will be surprised how quickly they will adjust.

Verbally respond

You can verbally reassure with shushing, humming, singing and using a 'broken record' technique, repeating the same sentence over and over. Maintain eye contact with your child. Even if the room is dark as outlined and they won't really be able to see you, be there emotionally. Focus on their face. Letting your child know that you are there will keep their stress levels low during times of upset. Looking at them can help them to process the change with your considered responses.

Lucy Says

The 'broken record' technique is repeating the same sentence over and over, for example 'It's sleep time, Harry, night night ...' Or you may find that singing a favourite song comforts your baby.

I am the first to acknowledge that these first two strategies can appear unhelpful. If your child is upset and crying, then touching them may irritate them and they will swat you away and not want you near them. Have some respect for that and reduce the touching. And if they are super upset they may not hear you, so now use the most effective tactic for settling – distraction.

Use distraction

Try to distract your child from crying. Crying and sleep are not related. Your child does not need to cry to go to sleep. The crying is a response to the changes you have made. It is typically a protest cry that goes in an up and down cycle. Your job is to bring the crying down into quiet so that then your child can start to fall asleep. This can sometimes happen rapidly; the child is very upset one moment and then asleep the next. I recommend distraction to help manage the crying wave and to help give your child moments of pause and calm. Although the crying-free moments may not last long, and your child may start crying again, introducing pockets of calm can make the stroking and rubbing more effective. For example:

- Gently blow on their face.
- Bang the bars of the cot or bang on the floor.
- Drum on the mattress.
- Use the white noise turned up loudly, then gradually turned down, then turned off (unless you plan to use it all night).
- Gently pat their chest to change the vibration of the crying.

Lucy Says

If you blow gently on your child's face, you will stop them in their tracks – they may stop and suck in their breath and in doing so present a pocket of calm within which the stroking and rubbing can be more effective as they can concentrate on the touch. They will start up again, but you are instrumental in helping them manage their level of upset.

These suggestions will not necessarily stop the crying, but they do help to manage the waves. You are being responsive and effective and supportive for this exercise. Many parents report that they would never think of this strategy as it doesn't necessarily fit with going to sleep, but keep in mind that your child is not going to go to sleep if they are crying. They need to self-regulate first and this can help.

The challenge of standing

Many children beyond the age of nine months will be able to stand up or pull themselves up, and dealing with this can be a barrier to getting them to go to sleep. I encourage parents to manage the situation and avoid getting into a power struggle.

If you teach your child how to be in the cot by staying down low on the floor, you can prevent this from becoming an issue. However, if standing is a problem, don't get into a power struggle – no one will win and very few children will go to sleep afterwards.

- During the day, get your child to practise going from standing to sitting to lying down.
- Use key words and phrases like 'lie down', 'all fall down'.
- Playing Ring-a-Rosy can help.
- During non-sleep time, show them how to run their hands down the cot bars to a sitting position.

Then, if they stand at bedtime/naptime or overnight:

- First allow them to get it out of their system. Let them do a lap of honour of the cot, then hug/comfort, put them down *once* and return to your low-down position.
- After that, if your child stands again, encourage them to come down on their own. Pat the mattress and stay down low on the floor yourself.
- Don't get into a power struggle.
- Wait for your child to come down themselves using your key words.
- At some point your child may get sleepy or dozy at the cotside while still standing. Then you can lie them down.

To pick up or not to pick up?

But can I pick them up? It's the million dollar question and one every parent wants to know the answer to. Most parents assume that the answer will be no, but ... *Of course you can pick them up to help them calm.*

Although I am not suggesting a pick up, put down approach as I feel it is too stimulating and unfair, especially if your child expects holding or rocking, I will always endorse picking up to prevent an indefinite cycle of crying. I would never want a child upset for an open-ended period of time, but I would also be conservative about picking up. I advise a pick up on a cycle of about 20–30 minutes.

Pick up the baby to calm them if they are hysterical. Stay and hold until calmer, but don't allow them to fall asleep in your arms.

I would like your child to come into a level of calm within 20–30 minutes of becoming upset. If possible, avoid picking up before this time frame. If you feel you must pick up, then absolutely do, but the more you pick up the longer it can take.

- Lift your child, shoulder cuddle, hold, rub, blow, comfort.
- Don't walk around or away from the cot.
- Once they have taken two or three calm breaths, return them to the cot.
- Resume your position and begin settling techniques again.
- Often the child can become more upset on returning to the cot. Avoid lifting them again immediately as you will perpetuate the cycle.
- Decide whether picking up helps.

Don't leave

Don't leave your child, or the bedroom, until they are asleep. Stay with your child until they are fast asleep. Don't leave the cot/bedside until they are breathing regularly – after ten minutes is normally safe. Do this at bedtime and during all night awakenings. Leaving too soon can wake them and make them hyper-vigilant.

Lucy Says

Now you know how to address the changes with the sleep learning exercise at bedtime, you need to have a plan for overnight. Addressing just bedtime in isolation will not normally resolve the nighttime activity, or it may take a very long time for the nights to improve. The overnight part of sleep also needs to be worked on. So after we have worked out the daytime structure we will look at the plan for overnight in Chapter 10.

Chapter 6

The Older Child:
Two and a half to six years

In this chapter we'll look at children aged between two and a half and six years old who are sleeping in a bed.

Sleep problems are not unique to infants and toddlers; they can linger well into the school-going age bracket. If your child has reached this stage and doesn't sleep well, you as parents may be resigned to the situation. I work with a high percentage of 'older children', which highlights that not all sleep difficulties just go away with time. Potentially, the older the child, the more difficult it can be to change long-ingrained habits and expectations. With age, the emotional landscape shifts as well, but the principles of healthy sleep practices already outlined still apply and your child's sleep *can always* be improved.

Of course, some children are better sleepers than others, and some children require more sleep and some a little less than the average, but all typically developing children are able to learn to go to sleep without a parent present or without delaying sleep for two or three hours at bedtime and to stay asleep overnight without wandering into the parents' bedroom or, indeed, looking for the parent to join them in their bed.

Quality sleep for your child should not be underestimated. It serves a far greater function than rest alone, contributing to optimised learning and mental alertness, increased ability to retain and process information and enhanced cognitive development.

When preschool and school-going children aged between two and a half and six years do not sleep well, the problems are normally either not being able to go to sleep easily at a reasonable time or not being able to stay asleep; and very often parental presence is required either at the onset of sleep or overnight, or both. Another common issue in this age range is staying awake for long periods of time overnight. Just as with younger children, in order for healthy sleep habits to develop and for your young child to be independent and efficient at sleeping, core elements apply. Positive sleep may be described as getting enough sleep for the age group, taking a daytime sleep when age-appropriate and/or required, the ability to go to sleep at a regular time and to be able to consolidate the nighttime sleep with minimum adult intervention.

How much sleep?

At age two and a half to six years your child may require 10–13 hours' sleep, including a nap if needed. Although by three years of age many children will no longer be napping – and many children will have stopped napping more than a year before they are biologically ready to do so – don't ever be afraid of reintroducing a nap (in the car, buggy, couch, for example) as you pick your way through their cycle of overtiredness. If your child will fall asleep on a journey in the car, then perhaps a nap may help. Plenty of parents report that if the child has a nap during the day they won't sleep until midnight, but that is just the deregulation of timing and not an indication that the nap is not needed or is unhelpful.

Chapter 8 details the best practice in feeding and sleeping for this age category, and you will be able to begin to apply all the principles previously outlined, along with the stay-and-support approach modified to suit a child in a bed.

Has your child stopped napping?

Although all children are different, it is usual for a child to nap until at least three years old, perhaps even closer to four. Some children 'give up' napping really early; others cling on for dear life. Very often a child who gives up really early may not be ready to give up that nap, but is resistant, and that makes us think that that is the reason. I like to see most children napping until *at least* two and a half years, in conjunction with routinely sleeping through the night, with the end of the nap being organic and not forced by parents or childcare.

As you already know, naps serve a vital function in mood, behaviour, eating and overnight sleeping patterns, so it is important that your child is offered a nap as long as they need it and to not rush them into stopping the naps. Eliminating the nap prematurely can often result in unwanted nighttime activity and early rising.

Here are some indicators that your child still needs to nap. If your child is under four years of age and:

1. They are tired at mid-morning/lunchtime.

2. They always fall asleep (in the car, for example) around the 1–2 p.m. mark.

3. They are really tired by 4–5 p.m.

4. They can't cope without a nap and have meltdowns in the evening.

5. They do not routinely sleep through the night.

When your child *is* ready to stop napping there are normally two different presentations. The first one may be that the nap starts to get shorter, shrinking from, say, two and a half hours to an hour or an hour and a half – and this would be age related. This indicates that the body needs less daytime sleep and that it is *preparing* not to nap at a time in the future.

You may find that your child starts refusing to nap or that before they are entirely ready to stop napping they start napping less frequently – taking a nap three days out of seven, for example. Again, this is the body preparing for the transition. It may be difficult to establish an exact nap need pattern, so keep providing the nap opportunity every day and encourage rest time even if the nap doesn't happen.

As your child makes this transition, from either the shrinking or the pacing perspective, you will need to start making further adjustments to ensure that the start of not napping does not cause bedtime resistance and/or frequent nighttime activity.

Between the ages of three and five years, the sleep amount recommendation endorsed by the American Academy of Sleep Medicine is from 10 to 13 hours. Once the nap element is gone the only way of achieving this quota is nighttime sleep. So make sure that you adjust bedtime forward to take account of the missing nap.

Lucy Says

If historically the single nap was for an hour and a half and bedtime was 8.30 p.m., without the nap bedtime may need to be at 7 p.m. to comfortably acclimatise the child to this new sleep pattern. Once this becomes established you may be able to move bedtime gradually back to 8.30 p.m.

Quiet time

Even without a nap, a toddler or pre-schooler may find it hard to get through the day without a break, so in the absence of a nap, allow for what I would describe as quiet time. Not necessarily in a bed, but on the couch and ideally no television. You could use reading or listening to audio books or music instead, and one hour would be the recommended duration, but to be honest anything would be helpful to ensure that they can get through the day until bedtime.

Even if you have had months of no naps, it would not be unusual for the nap to re-emerge for a while, especially as you improve the sleep situation. On that basis, allow it to happen, but don't allow the child to sleep past 2.30–3 p.m. or you may run the risk of bedtime being affected. With an occasional nap, plan for bedtime to occur about five hours after the nap, so begin preparations for the bedtime routine four hours and 15 minutes after the nap has finished. This way you always protect the bedtime process.

What is the right bedtime?

In this older age group bedtime may be from 7 p.m. to 9.30 p.m. and waking from 6 a.m. onwards, but in a lot of instances, a bedtime any later than 8 p.m. is simply too late, causing bedtime battles, frequent waking and shorter sleep duration. If you are struggling with your child's sleep, bringing forward bedtime will be an important element in the success of the plan, with or without a nap.

Consider the child's mood and behaviour in the evening. Many families report a poor mood or non-compliance, aggressive behaviour or just wanting to watch telly, and I suggest that this is all symptomatic of overtiredness. Even if your child's form is great in the evenings, make a clear decision to bring the timings forward in an effort to establish or re-establish positive sleep practices and in turn to identify your child's ideal bedtime. One of the only ways of ascertaining this is to bring the bedtime process forward *really* early, as I do with babies and toddlers, and then establish what bedtime should *actually* be. I call this 'landing bedtime'. For children who are coming from a 'sleep problem background', the actual time your child will sleep will likely be a lot earlier than you ever envisaged being possible.

When correcting the issues of older children we normally have five main jobs to do:

1. Decide whether naps are still required.

2. Establish an age-relevant bedtime.

3. Help them stay in bed with the new approach.

4. Help the child go to sleep with minimised parental input.

5. Diminish the cycle of waking overnight – this is perhaps the element that can take the longest.

The stay-and-support approach can be modified to take account of this and I am a big believer in giving the child an investment in their own sleep success and happiness. I create the right optics and I try to engage them and give them ownership and then in the background have the parent actively ingrain better sleep practices.

To start, you will need to observe the suggested daytime balance, with particular attention to the early onset of bedtime. I would also encourage you to participate in the activities outlined below, all of which help to package up the changes for your older child and enable you all to work towards positive sleep.

Elements to consider

The environment

Make sure your child's bedroom is a calm, safe place to be. Avoid too many distractions or stimulating activity in advance of sleep. Keep electronics and television out of the bedroom and restrict their use at least one or two hours before sleep time as using gadgets close to sleep can make it difficult for your child to switch off and have a restful sleep.

Exercise

Outdoor exercise and fresh air are a significant component in healthy sleep. At least one hour a day is the recommendation. Don't do this too close to sleep time, though, as in advance of sleep you need to help relax your child's body, not stimulate it.

Diet

As with everything in our lives, diet plays a large role in sleep. Your child will not sleep well if they are hungry. They need three structured meals a day and should be adequately hydrated throughout the day. Avoid high-sugar and processed foods. Dinner in the evening gives slow energy release and keeps the child going until morning. Allow two hours between eating and sleep to let the digestive system relax. Avoid vitamin supplements in the evening – if you do use them, give them early in the day. Consider foods that promote sleep, such as bananas, anything wholemeal and warm milk.

Sleep strategies

Talk to your child

Before you start, take your child aside and explain about the changes that you are planning to make. Don't do this at bedtime, do it during the day. Take them for a walk or talk over lunch and say that you are going to start a sleep learning exercise. Explain that you will help them learn to sleep better. If you currently stay with them when they are falling asleep, say that big girls or boys can do this solo. Explain that you will be staying with them to help them learn. Refer to a friend or relation they admire to help them through the process and have something to aim for. Avoid referring to siblings – this can add to a sense of displacement. Don't over talk the plan, but definitely put them on notice that changes are afoot.

Get your child involved

Let your child be involved in the decisions. It's a good idea to allow them to help you make the changes – rearrange the bedroom, change the orientation of the bed, perhaps purchase new items and give them a sense of ownership. If you have been bed hopping, start to close your bedroom door at night and encourage them to consider your room out of bounds; this will help them to define *their* place of sleep. I also think a picture of mum and dad in the bedroom is a nice idea to help them feel connected; and, if you were open to it, a parent's hand print on the wall next to their bed for them to match when they are going to sleep.

Create a bedtime zone

Create a bedtime zone in the bedroom. This is a space, other than the bed, where you carry out your new, improved bedtime routine. Often if your child relies on you to stay at bedtime, the bedtime routine and staying are merged together and I try to visually and physically make them two different activities. The bedtime zone is where you prepare for sleep and the bed is reserved for sleeping. The adult should never sit on the bed or lie down on the bed – this space is reserved for the child alone and *only* for sleeping.

To make the bedtime zone appealing, put down a rug and cushions, hang up a canopy, and perhaps some fairy lights; make this space *the* place to be. In this area you will go through your bedtime routine, have the chats and the cuddles; but when it is time for lights out, it will be time to climb into bed.

Define your new position

In preparation for implementing the sleep learning exercise, position a bean bag (as long as it's not a noisy one) or a cushion next to the bed for the parent to sit on when the lights go out and for if or when your child wakes overnight. As you proceed through the stages you will move the beanbag/cushion and this will be a visual and physical signal to the child that you are moving out of their sleep process.

Lucy Says

I firmly believe that how you package up the change dictates how successful the process will be – and not a reward chart in sight! I'm not against rewards charts but I do acknowledge, as a parent, that it can be very hard for *us* to be consistent with the reward system. In my own experience, my children couldn't care less about a star or minor reward after the first day or so – they just lose interest. Of course I do appreciate that there is a time and place to incentivise your child, but I will reserve that until closer to the end of the process and only when we have exhausted all other avenues!

Make a bedtime book

Although this may take some time, create a personal book of sleep to help illustrate the changes you are going to make and what you are hoping to achieve. Make it specific to your family, and use photos and text. Take pictures of your household – your kitchen, the bathroom, the cat, the bedroom. Show your child in words and in pictures the changes you are making and what you are working towards. Your child can help you make the book if you like, and allow them to keep the book in the bedroom, even under their pillow. They can show people when they visit and you can add to the book as time evolves.

Have a checklist for sleep

While you are being creative, also make a checklist to print off and stick on the wall in the bedtime zone to illustrate the steps of the bedtime routine.

For example:

- ☑ Brush teeth
- ☑ Wash hands
- ☑ Bedroom – get into pyjamas
- ☑ Read two stories
- ☑ Chat about the day
- ☑ Do sleep exercises
- ☑ Lights out

This small activity can really focus the young mind and is the 'to-do list' that you can check off as the bedtime routine unfolds. Some children with sleep difficulties want ultimate control and with this exercise we give it to them, but on our terms.

Set an alarm to start bedtime

If you feel that your child is resistant to starting the bedtime process, you are inclined to accede to requests for 'five more minutes', and it's hard to get going, set an alarm on your phone and offer a countdown to the alarm – when the alarm sounds we head off to the bedroom. If you use this strategy, you must do so with precision, otherwise its usefulness will diminish. It is a great limit-setting technique and helps to get bedtime moving.

Give them choices

I am big advocate of giving children choices. I found I had to become a skilled negotiator when I became a parent of a strong-willed child, and choices help defuse the complaints about not wanting to go to bed. I *never* ask a loaded question, like 'Do you want to go to bed?', 'Are you tired?' But I would ask *how* they want to go to bed: holding hands up the stairs; holding the bannister; what do they want to do first, teeth or hands?; what do they want to wear, the grey PJs or the blue ones?; which book are we reading, this one or that one?; what will we put on first, top or bottoms? This simple strategy helps take the focus off what your child *doesn't* want to do and what they *can* do. You can also have them make some of these decisions earlier in the day, like the PJs and the stories you will read.

Do role play

I also find that it helps if you spend some time role playing during non-sleep time what bedtime should look like. Your child can put their dolls or teddy bears to bed, simulating the process of bedtime. You are selling them the process – it's like a marketing exercise!

Lamp on a timer

If you can, I would recommend the use of a lamp on a timer for the bedtime routine. Set it to turn off after 20–30 minutes of the bedtime process. This is a great visual cue and you are not the instigator of the end of the process – the lamp is. When the light goes out, it's sleep time. You then escort your child to their bed, encourage them to climb in themselves and then, if you are weakening a dependency, apply the stay-and-support approach.

When you begin, it would not be unusual for your child to take *ages* to fall asleep, but this will improve with time. Remember, they are learning a new way to sleep.

Relaxation exercises

Make some relaxation and breathing exercises part of your bedtime routine. Breathing techniques and progressive muscle exercises can help the child learn how to relax their own body. They can do some with you and some without you being present. You could even create an illustrated guide using pictures of, for example, spaghetti, lemons or an elephant, so that your child can visualise the techniques too. You could make flash cards, together with your child, and use them as part of the bedtime routine, outside of the bed itself but in the bedtime zone.

☑ To start

- Take a deep breath in through your nose. Hold your breath for 6 seconds ... and now breathe out for 6 seconds.
- Take another deep breath through your nose and imagine your tummy is a big balloon filling up with air.
- Hold your breath for 6 seconds ... now breathe out for 6 seconds and imagine that the air in the balloon is slowly escaping.

☑ Legs

- Stretch out your legs in front of you and point your toes. Squeeze the muscles in the top of your legs ... now squeeze the muscles in the bottom of your legs ... hold it. Now relax ... let your legs go limp.
- Imagine that your legs are floppy cooked spaghetti and relax all the muscles in your legs.
- Be aware of how your legs feel.
- Now take a deep breath, filling that balloon, and hold for 6 seconds ... and breathe out for 6 seconds.

☑ Hands

- Make a fist with your left hand and squeeze tight. Imagine that you are holding an orange and you are squeezing all the juice out of the orange ... hold it tight ... and now relax your hand.
- Be aware of how your hand feels.
- Now make a fist with your right hand and squeeze tight. Imagine that you are holding a lemon and squeezing all the juice out. Feel the tightness in your hand and arm ... hold it ... and now relax your hand.
- Now take a deep breath, filling the balloon, and hold for 6 seconds ... and breathe out for 6 seconds.

☑ Arms

- Stretch your arms out in front of you as if you're reaching for something ... keep stretching ... hold it ... and relax.
- Let your arms drop to your sides. Imagine your arms, like your legs, are spaghetti hanging at your sides. Relax your arms.
- Be aware of how your arms feel.
- Now stretch your arms up above your head ... try to reach for the sky with your fingertips ... hold ... keep reaching ... now let your arms drop to your sides ... relax your arms ... let your arms go very loose.
- Now take a deep breath, filling the balloon, and hold for 6 seconds ... and breathe out for 6 seconds.

☑ Shoulders

- Pull your shoulders up to your ears ... hold ... keep holding ... now relax.
- Now take a deep breath, filling the balloon, and hold for 6 seconds ... and breathe out for 6 seconds.

☑ Tummy

- Pull in your tummy muscles. Imagine that an elephant has just stepped on your tummy ... suck in all the muscles in your tummy ... hold it ... now relax.

- Let your stomach out ... relax all the muscles in your tummy.
- Now take a deep breath, filling the balloon, and hold for 6 seconds ... and breathe out for 6 seconds.

☑ Face

- Screw up your face as much as you can. Wrinkle your nose ... mouth ... eyes ... forehead ... cheeks ... and purse your lips together ... hold it ... now relax.
- Let all the muscles in your face go limp.
- Now take a deep breath, filling the balloon, and hold for 6 seconds ... and breathe out for 6 seconds.

☑ Relax

- Now relax your whole body. Imagine you're a rag doll and try to relax all the muscles in your body. Notice how relaxed and calm you feel.
- Now take a deep breath, filling the balloon, and hold for 6 seconds ... and breathe out for 6 seconds.

Well done!

The children I work with love this routine. It puts a new slant on bedtime and helps to serve an important relaxation function too.

The anxious child

A newly discovered or, indeed, pre-existing fear of the dark, scary thoughts and nightmares are usual in young children. Commonly, from two years of age, as your child develops a greater sense of self their imagination and creativity blossom. This can sometimes lead to a resistance at bedtime and not wanting to be left alone when the lights go out. Your child may become scared of their bedroom and demand parental presence both at bedtime and when they wake overnight and this may be challenging to manage, especially if the this behaviour suddenly emerges out of nowhere, which it can.

First of all, it is a normal part of development. It is usually just a phase and it is important that we give weight to the situation, but that we don't allow the young child, over time, to use their fear and anxiety as a stalling tactic where bedtime is concerned. Our task as parents is to help our children feel loved, safe and secure.

Nightmares, fears and anxieties are common in young children, and scary dreams usually occur in the second part of the night during REM or 'dreaming' sleep. At least one in four children aged three to six years report having perhaps one nightmare a week. This can be very alarming for a young child and the fear is very real. Typical nightmares involve being chased or stuck somewhere. Your child will require reassurance and comfort from you during and after a nightmare.

Being afraid of the dark can also emerge, without any triggers; you may recall as a child yourself being uncomfortable or fearful in the dark and imagining monsters under the bed, ready to grab you as you get in or out of the bed – I know I do. If you as an adult are still not comfortable in the dark, try not to project this onto your child.

Some ideas that may help:

☑ Ensure that the bedroom is a calm and sleep-inducing environment with a night light so that it is not pitch black. Try not to allow lamps and big lights, such as hall or bathroom lights, to be left on as they may interfere with the onset of sleep and make staying asleep more challenging. Choose night lights instead, or use a string of fairy lights to illuminate the room. I love the battery-operated dimming fairy light strings, as they are super bright at the start and gradually get dimmer. This and can help ease your child into not being afraid of the dark.

☑ Make sure that the bed is cosy and comfortable. Some children will feel more secure if the bed is placed next to a wall and they have a bed rail so that they are enclosed.

☑ Avoid bringing your child out of their bedroom and into other rooms in the house when they express fear; comfort and support them in their bedroom so that you don't ingrain room anxiety.

☑ Spend lots of non-sleep time in the room with them, play with them and dress them in the bedroom for at least 30 minutes per day.

☑ If you haven't already, give your child a security item. Persuade your child that the stuffed toy or doll will help him or her to be brave and will help keep them safe too. You could also give your child the task of looking after the item so that they are in charge and have a task to take their mind off their worries.

☑ Consider a wand or a shield to help your child feel empowered. While you don't want to validate the fear, making your child think that there really is something to be afraid of, you do want them to develop coping mechanisms that can help them overcome their fears and anxieties.

☑ If your child is afraid of the dark, help them to learn to have fun in the dark by playing games during non-sleep time, with the lights out, possibly with torches. If your child is very resistant to this, you could start the games in bright light and gradually turn the lights down as they get more comfortable.

☑ It would be wise to avoid inadvertently exposing your child to scary or frightening images, programmes or audio. Sometimes overhearing the radio news in the car can unsettle children who have a tendency to be anxious and fearful.

☑ Pick with care the type of books that you read at bedtime and be mindful of anything that may cause fear and anxiety in the young mind.

☑ Talk openly to your child about what disturbs them. Do this during the day rather than at bedtime. Set aside a time each day for this exercise. Never make fun of their fear, but encourage them to overcome it by taking control of how they feel. Writing out or drawing pictures and then throwing them away can help.

☑ Increase time spent with your child. What most children really crave is parental attention. Allow for 10–20 minutes one-to-one time, led by your child.

☑ Encourage your child to take control of a scary dream by choosing how it ends. Let them be the director of the dream or of their worrying thoughts – they could bring in a super hero to save the day, for example. Doing this helps dissolve the fear factor and change scary into fun.

☑ Try not to feed their fears by searching the house for monsters; instead explain that you will keep them safe and that the bedroom is a positive place to be. Some parents report that a 'monster spray' – just water in a spray bottle – helping to ward off bad thoughts is a great help.

☑ Develop further coping mechanisms for any scary thoughts or inability to fall asleep easily. You could use additional breathing exercises and/or some visualisations that can be done without parent(s).

Additional breathing exercises to do when lying in bed:

1. Take two slow breaths: in through the nose and out through the mouth.

2. Imagine the air flow travelling through one nostril and out through the other. Then reverse this pattern.

3. Concentrating on breathing can help a child focus and avoid distractions. If they don't fall asleep with this method, it will clear the way for sleep to happen.

Visualisations:

1. Get your child to select some pictures of fun things to do or nice place to be, like a funfair or a beach, from a catalogue or online.

2. Let them take one picture at sleep time and use this to create a relaxing, fear-free story that they can direct while lying in bed before falling asleep.

Gentle stretching exercises:

1. Lie flat on the bed.

2. Point the toes of your right foot as far as they can go.

3. Hold for four seconds and release.

4. Do the same with the left foot.

5. Then do the same with hands/arms.

6. Practise this with the breathing routine mentioned above.

The bedtime routine

Establish a bedtime routine in your child's bedroom, allocating 20–30 minutes to help your child become quiet and relaxed. Be creative and loving; indulge in plenty of physical contact. Gentle massage, stretching and relaxing exercises. Cuddles and stories. Chatting about the day and what you are looking forward to doing tomorrow. Use music or audio books during the wind-down, but turn them off before sleep time. Consider meditation for children if your young child finds it difficult to switch off.

Make sure that you have an end to the bedtime routine – the lamp timer will help. Common issues here involve delaying tactics, calling you back after you have left the room: hunger, pain, not tired, scared, need a wee-wee. Try to meet the objections in advance and don't fall victim to giving into demands for extra drinks, toilet runs (within reason) or one more story. A pre-sleep ritual can set the scene for lights out and sleep time. You may even need a few guidelines, such as 'Once the lights go out, no talking ... close your eyes ... go to sleep.'

Lucy Says

Now you will either leave as you normally do or you will sit next to the bed and use the stay-and-support approach. If you typically leave and your child follows you, return them to the bed at least once. If they follow you again or are upset when you leave a second time, return to the room and then commit to staying to break the cycle of getting in and out of the bed. Help them learn to stay in the bed with your presence.

Chapter 7

Feeding and Sleeping Suggestions: Birth to six months

T he following pages outline feeding and sleeping suggestions from the early days to six months. Don't come home from the hospital and immediately implement this advice; give yourself time to adjust and then at six weeks onwards you might like to start seeing what is effective for you. You can start this at any stage and age; just work within the age-relevant suggestions for your baby. These suggestions should never be applied rigidly; in the early months they should be viewed only as a framework.

Up to two months

Expectations

- Total amount of sleep: 14–17 hours in a 24-hour period.
- Number of naps: five to eight throughout the day.
- Daytime sleep not necessarily organised, with naps being anything from 40 minutes to two or three hours per sleep segment.

- Don't worry about nap lengths; get the balance between the naps working well and the natural duration may emerge in time.
- Feeds: every three hours for bottle-fed babies, possibly more frequent for breastfed babies.
- Feeds will be on a 24-hour basis, with some possibility of longer stretches in the overnight period as time passes.

Review your feeding practice

BREASTFEEDING

It is possible that your breastfed baby will require more frequent feeds, especially as you establish your feeding practice. Prioritise your supply and technique before worrying about following a routine, but once mum and baby are in sync then you can start to set some additional landmarks in the day.

As a breastfeeding mum myself, I really encourage mums to try and persevere with breastfeeding. It's helpful to attend a breastfeeding class before your baby is born and then seek support, if needed, from that consultant in the early days as you establish feeding. It can be challenging, not to mention toe-curlingly painful at the start, but very much worth pursuing, if you can. As time evolves, it is worth considering making sure that you don't teach your baby to graze all day and in turn all night. A negative feeding cycle can emerge, which can cause much pain (sore nipples) and upset for all involved and even result in many mums giving up breastfeeding early.

Once feeding is established, work towards feeding every two to three hours so that the feeds are adequate, your supply is maintained and your feed time and sleep time don't continually clash and start to cause a feed and sleep difficulty.

Lucy Says

Don't let other people undermine you when your breastfed baby is unsettled. It is unlikely that your

feeding method will be the reason why your baby
is fussy or doesn't sleep for long, although this may
be suggested. A bottle of formula is not always the
answer. Be confident and follow your instincts – you
can have a healthy breastfed baby who sleeps – these
two activities are not mutually exclusive. I breastfed all
four of my children and they slept well too!

Once your breastfeeding is established, I also suggest that you should introduce a bottle, not necessarily of formula, but of expressed milk, from six weeks onwards, in order to avoid bottle refusal later on. The last thing I would want to do is undermine your breastfeeding relationship with what may described as nipple confusion, but many babies, if they are not offered a bottle early on, refuse a bottle later, which can cause untold stress and anxiety for parents, especially if you are heading back to work. Or it can mean that mum feels trapped by being the only one that can attend to the baby as they get older, leaving the mum, and possibly those around her, want to discontinue breastfeeding. Introducing a bottle once a day helps avoid this. Also, it can be another way of mum getting some solid sleep in the early months. The other parent can provide the last feed, with mum heading to bed early before the middle of the night feed is due.

Lucy Says

I probably would not have survived the early months,
especially when I had more than one child, without
going to bed at 7–8 p.m. and allowing dad to provide
a bottle of expressed milk at 10–11 p.m. This way,
my next feed was at 1–2 a.m. (or later if I was lucky)
and I had already potentially had five or six hours of
unbroken sleep, which is very helpful for everyone in
the family. Self care is paramount in the early months.

BOTTLE FEEDING

If you have decided to bottle feed or, for whatever reason, your breastfeeding has been unsuccessful, don't feel that you have failed. How you feed your baby is a personal choice and I dislike the culture of 'us and them'. I was lucky to have a positive breastfeeding experience with all my children, but would never be inclined to feel superior on that basis or undermine a parent who is bottle feeding. Basically, we are all just doing the best we can for and with our children – that is what matters.

Ensure that you are preparing your bottle feeds as outlined by the manufacturer and that your baby is being offered the correct amount of milk at each feed time. Find the right teat and make sure that over time you adjust to increase the milk flow and avoid frustration. Similarly, don't let your baby to drink on a drip-feed basis over the course of a few hours. Once your baby is established on bottles, provide a feed for about 40 minutes and then move to the next feed time so you don't create a negative feed cycle, impaired appetite and unnecessary wind.

Make sure that during and after each feed, your baby is winded correctly so that this does not start to cause a problem.

Feeding and sleeping suggestions

7–7.30 a.m.	Start the day no later than 7.30 a.m., regardless of what has happened overnight
	Get out of bed and expose your baby to natural/bright light
	Provide a morning feed within the first 30 minutes of waking to anchor your day feeds, regardless of what feeds have happened overnight
7.45–9 a.m.	Prepare for your first nap within 45 minutes and no longer than 1½ hours of being awake
	Pay attention to your baby's sleep cues and act on them
	If you don't see them looking tired, prepare for the nap 10–20 minutes before the end of the suggested wake period
	This nap may be as short as 40 minutes or it may be more than an hour

	Allow your baby to wake naturally, but wake them to maintain your next feed, which will be due three hours after the first morning feed
10–10.30 a.m.	Provide a feed Expose to natural light Leisure time
11 a.m.–12 p.m.	Depending on time and duration of Nap 1, prepare for the next nap within 1½–2 hours of being awake Be careful not to plan your sleep time according to the time your baby has fed – base it on the time your baby woke and also read their sleep cues This nap may be as short as 40 minutes or it may be more than an hour Allow your baby to wake naturally, but wake them to maintain your next feed, which will be due three hours after the second morning feed
1–1.30 p.m.	Provide a feed Expose to natural light Leisure time
2–3 p.m.	Within 1½–2 hours of waking, baby should be asleep again Read their sleep cues but don't allow them to stay awake longer than this suggested time frame
4–4.30 p.m.	Provide a feed Expose to natural light Leisure time
5–6 p.m.	Asleep again within 1½–2 hours of waking
7–7.30 p.m.	Feed
7.30–11 p.m.	May nap on and off until your bedtime, with a last feed around 10/11 p.m. and feed then throughout the night as needed until morning Your baby's bedtime is quite late at the start but will get earlier as the first few months pass It is likely that you will keep your baby with you until then, sleeping on you or in a Moses basket/ pram close to you until you go to bed Prepare for bed no more than 1½ hours after the last nap

Take your baby to the bedroom and provide the nighttime feed and when you are ready start using the percentage of wakefulness concept as your baby is going to sleep

Provide nighttime feeds as required

Keep the night feed in the bedroom and be as non-stimulating as possible

Lucy Says

I want to stress that all babies are different and imposing a strict routine on your baby may not be appropriate or necessary; this guide should be implemented with flexibility, keeping in mind safe sleep recommendations and primarily ensuring that your child is getting enough to drink and gaining weight accordingly.

Lucy's checklist

☑ Be very careful not to over-stimulate or allow your baby to get overtired by staying awake too long. Some babies can only manage 45 minutes' wakefulness at the start of the day; this typically gets longer as the day goes on, with one and a half to a maximum of two hours of waking time at any one time.

☑ Get to know your baby. Not every cry means that they are hungry. Have a checklist – hungry, tired, cold, bored, nappy change, for example.

☑ Keep in mind that some babies need more assistance than others and really do need your help to settle. 'Self-soothing' skills may not become possible for another few months. In the interim, make sure that you facilitate the sleep process by observing all the other elements outlined.

☑ Beyond six weeks, start to create a consistent bedtime routine to set up the right sleep cues for baby. Understanding what happens next can make the transition from awake to asleep almost seamless for your baby.

☑ Focus on bedtime, which will probably be quite late. Be conscious of sleep habits and patterns and work on putting your baby into bed relaxed but awake, using the percentage of wakefulness concept. Stay nearby and soothe gently as they finish off falling asleep. Physically comfort and support them as they develop the ability.

☑ If it doesn't feel right, stop and try again at a later date.

☑ Know that it takes longer to establish daytime sleep, so napping can be disorganised until six months plus.

☑ Most babies benefit from three to eight naps of varied duration during wake windows of 45 minutes to two hours throughout the day until bedtime, and three-hourly feeds.

☑ Many naps may still be short, about 40–45 minutes, but will gradually lengthen if the baby is getting enough sleep and becoming more independent, capable and efficient at falling asleep.

☑ At the end of month two, and definitely by the end of month three you should probably begin to phase out motion sleep in cars/swings for Nap 1 and Nap 2 and get them sleeping in the Moses basket or cot, depending on what you are using. The rest of the day sleeps can be motion-oriented.

Lucy Says

During the early months some babies will sleep better than others – all babies can eventually become great sleepers in time and especially within the second half of the first year. Parents may find the early months draining and exhilarating all at the same time, but don't worry. Longer stretches of sleep are just around the corner.

Two to four months

Your baby's sleep is getting more organised. You may see some longer stretches of sleep, but don't worry if you are not. You may be sick of hearing it, but all babies are different and if you follow my advice you are setting a firm foundation for good sleep practices and ensuring that *your* baby reaches *their* optimum amounts of sleep. Once you get beyond four months, if things are still varied your child will be a little more robust and you may consider working more intensively on your child's sleep ability.

Expectations

- Total amount of sleep: 10½–12 hours overnight/with feeds.
- Total amount of daytime sleep: four to five hours.
- Number of naps: three to six, depending on wake time and nap duration.
- Daytime sleep will be becoming more organised, with naps being anything from 40 minutes to two or three hours per sleep segment.
- Don't worry about nap lengths; get the balance between the naps working well and the duration will emerge in time.
- Feeds: every three hours during the day, possibly longer overnight.
- Nighttime feeds may still be appropriate until closer to nine months of age.

Review your feeding practice

I would anticipate that your feeding practice is now established and that you are comfortably feeding more or less on a three-hourly basis through the day and possibly longer overnight, if you are lucky! If your baby is still waking frequently overnight, that is perfectly normal. Make sure that you are observing all the other recommendations from Chapter 4 and this will diminish in time. Your young baby will still require a number of nighttime feeds, anything from every three hours plus from bedtime onwards, until they start to get a bit older, but by around four months you may really see a pattern emerge. Although I appreciate that it would be great if the night feeds diminished as early as possible, please understand that night feeds may remain until at least nine months and we just have to meet that need. It is our task as parents.

ALLOW TO WAKE OR DREAM FEED?

Now that bedtime will be commencing earlier you may be thinking about how best to manage the nighttime feeds. There are lots of schools of thought on this and I have to say that I am not a fan of the dream feed. To clarify, a dream or sleepy feed is where the parent initiates the nighttime feed at a certain time – normally between 10 p.m. and 11.30 p.m. – when the child is still asleep. The baby is lifted and provided a feed in the hope that it will 'see them through' until morning. For some, this is effective and does exactly that. However, I see a large number of babies who are being woken for a dream feed but who then go on to wake frequently and additional feeds are provided. The feeds may be needed, but perhaps the dream feed is not, and the very act of initiating the feed is disrupting your child's inner rhythm, which makes the dream feed counter-productive. I personally advocate a feed when your baby wakes, provided this is within a reasonable time of the last feed. This way the feed is baby-led and supported by you and there is a higher possibility that parents will reach a reduced or no night feed territory sooner – if your baby is biologically ready.

I also would *not* suggest cool boiled water as a milk feed substitute. There is no rush to make your child sleep through when they still require a feed. Make all the other adjustments and the feeds will go away when your child is biologically able. If this does not emerge after nine months, you can start observing a night weaning exercise, detailed later.

Feeding and sleeping suggestions

Wake time	6–7.30 a.m.	Start the day no later than 7.30 a.m., regardless of what has happened overnight
		Get out of bed and expose your baby to natural/bright light
		Provide a morning feed within the first 30 minutes of waking to anchor your day feeds, regardless of what feeds have happened overnight
Nap 1	7.00–9.30 a.m.	Prepare for your first nap within 1–2 hours of being awake
		Pay attention to your baby's sleep cues and act on them
		If you don't see them looking tired, prepare for the nap 20 minutes before the end of the suggested wake period
		This nap may be as little as 40 minutes or it may be an hour or more
		Allow your baby to wake naturally, but wake them to maintain your next feed, which will be due three hours after the first morning feed
Awake	9–10.30 a.m.	Provide a feed within three hours of the morning feed. The timing will depend on the morning feed time
		Expose to natural light
		Leisure time
Nap 2	10.30–12 p.m.	Depending on time and duration of Nap 1, prepare for the next nap within 1½–2 hours of being awake
		Be careful not to plan your sleep time according to the time your baby has fed – base it on the time your baby woke and also read their sleep cues
		This nap may be as short as 40 minutes or it may be more than an hour
		Allow your baby to wake naturally, but wake them to maintain your next feed, which will be due three hours after the second morning feed
Awake	1.30–2.30 p.m.	Provide a feed within three hours of the last feed
		Expose to natural light
		Leisure time

Naps 3/4/5	3–4 p.m.	Depending on time and duration of Nap 2, provide a third/fourth/fifth nap as required within 1½–2 hours of being awake
		Your baby will then be awake from 4.30 to 6 p.m. at the latest and the next sleep will be bedtime, which will gradually get earlier, to anywhere between 6 and 8 p.m., depending on when the last nap finishes
	4.30–5.30 p.m.	Provide a feed within three hours of the last feed
		Consider a cluster or split feed so that you can provide a feed closer to bedtime
	6.15–7.15 p.m.	Prepare for bed about 1¼–1½ hours after the final nap
		Provide the bath and/or bedtime routine
		Provide the bedtime feed (or remainder of)
		Operate the percentage of wakefulness approach
Sleep	6.30–8 p.m.	Within 1¼–1½ hours of the last nap, prepare for bedtime
		Provide the remainder of the last feed and begin your bedtime routine, ideally using the percentage of wakefulness approach
Bedtime	6/7.30 a.m.	Your baby will still require nighttime feed(s)
		Your baby may sleep for longer stretches, but still be wakeful in the later part of the night as you head towards morning
		Provide feeds accordingly and comfort and support as needed

Lucy's checklist

☑ During this time frame you may start to see night sleep being more organised, and you can begin to concentrate on the quality and quantity of your child's sleep: the amount of sleep they get and the place where they sleep.

☑ There is a natural variation in how long babies of this age can sleep. Some will sleep more than others – this is just the way it is.

☑ By now I would strongly advise that you avoid allowing

baby to graze or snack all day or they'll get into the habit and transfer this requirement into the nighttime period as well; most babies who are breast and bottle fed can go three hours between feeds.

☑ Feed in quiet places with few distractions so that they can concentrate on the feed and satisfy their hunger.

☑ If you want your child to sleep in their Moses basket/cot, try to avoid bringing them into your bed during the night. Return them to the cot after their nighttime feed to avoid an expectation of bed-sharing if you can't or don't want to commit to that as a family.

☑ At the end of month three and definitely by the end of month four you should probably phase out motion sleep in cars/swings for Nap 1 and Nap 2 and get them sleeping in the Moses basket or cot, depending on what you are using. The rest of the day naps can be motion-oriented.

☑ Be mindful of your baby's growth spurts and milestones that can disturb sleep. The Wonder Weeks app is a useful guide for checking whether these are the reasons for any regressions.

☑ Towards the four-month mark your baby is developing a better body clock and may be able to stay awake for longer periods, but you really need to avoid them getting overtired, fussy and hard to settle as this will negatively impact their nighttime sleep. Two hours of wakefulness is still a good guide.

☑ Neurologically the character of your baby's sleep is evolving and locking into place. Be mindful of what your baby associates with falling asleep and try to allow them to perfect the skill of falling asleep at bedtime, continuing to reduce parental input. If this task has been impossible, you may just need to resign yourself to it for a while longer and then from six months onwards begin to learn about my effective stay-and-support approach.

Four to six months

Expectations

- Total amount of nighttime sleep: 10–12 hours with or without feed(s), depending on the child,
- Nighttime feeds may still be appropriate until closer to nine months of age.
- Total amount of daytime sleep: three to four hours.
- Number of naps: three to five.
- Feeds: three- to four-hourly, with or without solid food (as you decide).
- Suggested milk need: 1050ml in a 24-hour period and/or breastfeeds.

Lucy Says

I would anticipate a daytime sleep need in the region of three to four hours, balanced between three or four naps, maybe even five. Some children in this age group, if they are having two very good naps, might have only three naps per day, but many will still need four to five naps throughout the day. This will reduce in time.

If you are breastfeeding I would encourage you to work towards three- to four-hourly feeds now, never in an effort to make your child hungry, but to encourage the feed and sleep rhythm to run in sync. If you feel your baby requires more frequent breastfeeds, do provide them, but try to do this midway between sleeps as opposed to always just before nap time.

Introducing solid foods

It is not recommended that you introduce solid foods before at least six months; however, all children are different and many parents decide, either themselves or with their healthcare practitioner, to introduce solid food before this time. This is an informed decision to be made yourself, with your GP or health nurse, bearing in mind that the World Health Organization suggests waiting until the child is at least six months. I wouldn't be inclined to start solid food early with the anticipation that it will improve sleep – this rarely happens. Whenever you begin the solid food/weaning process, be sure to follow a plan, baby-led or otherwise, and then introduce meals at the times I advise. I don't think it's a good idea to begin solid food and your work on sleep on the same day; pace both so that you can see what is having a positive (or negative) impact.

Feeding and sleeping suggestions

Wake time First feed Breakfast*	6–7.30 a.m.	From 6 a.m., and no later than 7.30 a.m., get up and start the day
		Provide first feed within the first half hour and breakfast (if applicable) within the next half hour
		Wake your child by 7.30 a.m. if still asleep to regulate body clock regardless of what has happened overnight
Nap 1 – cot	8–9.30 a.m.	This nap should start within 1½–2 hours of waking
		Follow your child's sleep cues or prepare for this nap 20 minutes before the end of the suggested wake time
		This nap can be at least 45 minutes to one hour+ in duration
		Allow to wake naturally or wake after 1½ hours maximum
Awake/leisure time Second feed Lunch*	10–11.30 a.m.	Between the first and second nap, provide the second feed, and lunch if applicable
		The time will depend on wake time and nap duration
		There is a 1½–2-hour window of wakefulness after Nap 1 ends and before Nap 2 needs to start

		Feed and lunch should be over in time for the nap
		Follow your child's sleep cues or prepare for the nap 20 minutes before the end of the suggested waking period
Nap 2 – cot	11 a.m.–12.30 p.m.	Start time of Nap 2 depends on Nap 1 start time and duration
		Your child should be put down within 1½–2 hours of waking from Nap 1
		Pay attention to sleep signals
		Nap 2 will ideally be 1 hour+ in duration
		Allow to wake naturally or wake to keep your next feed time in place
Awake/leisure time	2–3 p.m.	Provide feed within 4 hours of the previous feed
Third feed		This should happen after Nap 2
Naps 3, 4, 5 – car/buggy	3–4 p.m.	Depending on time and duration of Nap 2, provide further naps as required within 1½–2 hours of waking from the previous nap
		Duration: 10 minutes – 1 hour+
		Allow to wake naturally or wake by 4.30/5 p.m. at the latest
		These naps can be on the go in the car, buggy or sling; not the cot as it can be too difficult for most babies
Dinner time*	5–5.30 p.m.	Provide dinner if applicable.
Final feed	6–6.15 p.m.	Provide bedtime feed
		Do this away from the bedroom, with the lights on, so that it has nothing to do with sleep
		Ensure a clear 45 minutes between feed end and sleep time
Bedtime routine	6.20–6.30 p.m.	Start bath (if doing one) and/or the bedtime routine in the bedroom where your child will sleep

Into cot	6.50 p.m.	Place your child in the cot/use the percentage of wakefulness approach as required
Aim to be asleep	7 p.m.	Aim for the child to be asleep, maintaining no more than a 2-hour window of wakefulness between the end of the last nap and being in bed asleep

Solid food if established

Lucy Says

Children wake up overnight – it is a biological fact.

Your child will wake less often and will sleep with little intervention when they are not hungry or uncomfortable.

There is no 'normal'; it is your child's sleep *ability* that we are enhancing.

Chapter 8

Feeding and Sleeping Suggestions: Six months to six years

Over the next few pages I am going to outline my age-appropriate feeding and sleeping suggestions from six months to six years of age. When you have reviewed your child's age group, proceed to the next chapter so that you can get a feel of how to develop the routine to apply and why each application has merit and method so that you honour the balance as it is meant to be applied.

Six to eight months

Expectations

- Total amount of nighttime sleep: 10–12 hours with or without a feed, depending on the child.
- Nighttime feeds may still be appropriate until closer to nine months of age.
- Total amount of daytime sleep: 3–3½ half hours.
- Number of naps: three.
- Feeds: four-hourly, with solid food as appropriate.

- Suggested milk need six–seven months: 960ml in four feeds and/or breastfeeds.
- Suggested milk need seven–eight months: 630ml in three feeds and/or breastfeeds. (The feed that is dropped first is the mid-morning one; replace with meat protein.)

Lucy Says

I would anticipate a daytime sleep need in the region of three to three and a half hours, balanced between three naps. Some children in this age group, if they are having two very good naps, might have only two naps per day, but the majority of babies will benefit from this biologically appropriate third nap until closer to eight months and they are sleeping well both by day and at night.

If you are breastfeeding I would encourage you to work towards four-hourly feeds now, never in an effort to make your child hungry, but to encourage the feed and sleep rhythm to run in sync. If you feel your baby requires more frequent breastfeeds, do provide them, but try to do this midway between sleeps as opposed to always just before nap time.

Introducing solid foods

Solid food is generally introduced from six months onwards; you will start with small tastes, ideally following a plan, and then graduate to meat protein by seven to eight months as advised by your GP or health nurse. At the early stages, the milk is more important than the food, so don't allow the solid food to overpower the feeds. By the time your child is nine months plus, solid food will start to be more important and the milk need is shrinking, so that by the time your child is twelve months the milk need will have shrunk to 240–420ml per day and your child will have three solid meals and two to three healthy snacks as appropriate.

Feeding and sleeping suggestions

Wake time First feed Breakfast	6–7.30 a.m.	From 6 a.m., and no later than 7.30 a.m., get up and start the day Provide first feed within the first half hour and breakfast (if applicable) within the next half hour Wake your child by 7.30 a.m. if still asleep to regulate body clock regardless of what has happened overnight
Nap 1 – cot	8–9.30 a.m.	This nap should start within 1½–2 hours of waking Follow your child's sleep cues or prepare for this nap 20 minutes before the end of the suggested wake time This nap can be at least 45 minutes to one hour+ in duration Allow to wake naturally or wake after 1½ hours maximum
Awake/leisure time Second feed Lunch	10–11.30 a.m.	Between the first and second nap, provide the second feed and lunch The time will depend on wake time and nap duration There is a 2–3-hour window of wakefulness after Nap 1 ends and before Nap 2 needs to start Feed and lunch should be over in time for the nap Follow your child's sleep cues or prepare for the nap 20 minutes before the end of the suggested waking period Note that around 7 months onwards this milk feed is replaced with meat protein introduction
Nap 2 – cot	11 a.m.–12.30 p.m.	Start time of Nap 2 depends on Nap 1 start time and duration Your child should be put down within 2–3 hours of waking from Nap 1 Pay attention to sleep signals

		Nap 2 will ideally be 1 hour+ in duration
		Allow to wake naturally or wake to keep your next feed time in place
Awake/leisure time Third feed and snack	2–3 p.m.	Feed time/healthy snack time (depending on the previous feed) should happen after Nap 2
Nap 3 – car/ buggy	3–4 p.m.	Depending on time and duration of Nap 2, provide a third nap within 1½–2 hours of waking Nap 3 can be 10 minutes to 1 hour+ in duration Allow to wake naturally or wake by 4.30/5 p.m. at the latest This nap can be on the go in the car, buggy or sling; not the cot as it can be too difficult for most babies
Dinner time	5–5.30 p.m.	Provide dinner – protein and carbohydrate – when established
Final feed	6–6.15 p.m.	Provide bedtime feed Do this away from the bedroom, with the lights on, so that it has nothing to do with sleep Ensure a clearance of 45 minutes between end of feed and sleep time
Bedtime routine	6.20–6.30 p.m.	Start bath (if doing one) and/or the bedtime routine in the bedroom where your child will sleep
Into cot	6.50 p.m.	Place your child in the cot/use the stay-and-support approach as required
Aim to be asleep	7 p.m.	Aim for your child to be asleep, maintaining not more than a 2–2½-hour window of wakefulness between the end of the last nap and being in bed asleep If the final nap finished early, bring bedtime forward to accommodate this

Eight to twelve months

Expectations

- Total amount of nighttime sleep: 10½–12 hours.
- From nine months (or before), night feeds generally not required.
- Total amount of daytime sleep: 2½–3 hours.
- Number of naps: two.
- Feeds: three per day, 630ml and/or breastfeeds.
- Milk need will decrease further as your baby gets closer to 12 months.
- Three solid meals/two to three healthy snacks/meat protein.

Lucy Says

I would anticipate a daytime sleep need in the region of two and a half to three hours, balanced between two naps. Some children in this age group, if their two main naps are not long enough, will benefit from a third in the car or buggy, which should be over by 4.30 p.m. at the latest to prevent overtiredness at bedtime.

A word about milk feeds

I would anticipate that your child now requires three milk feeds per day with a recommended amount of 630ml and that the feeds are only given during waking hours, not at night. I would also recommend three meals with meat protein, specifically in the evening. Don't worry if your child's milk consumption is more or less; as we work on your child's sleep you can increase or reduce as required, bearing in mind that by 12 months the milk need shrinks further and solid food is king. If you find that your child drinks more milk than advised and in turn is a fussy eater, these adjustments will help.

Feeding and sleeping suggestions

Wake time First feed Breakfast	6–7.30 a.m.	From 6 a.m., and no later than 7.30 a.m., get up and start the day Provide first feed within the first half hour and breakfast within the next half hour Wake your child by 7.30 a.m. if still asleep to regulate body clock regardless of what has happened overnight
Nap 1 – cot	8–9.30 a.m.	This nap should start within 2 hours of waking Follow your child's sleep cues or prepare for this nap 20 minutes before the end of the suggested wake time This nap can be at least 45 minutes to 1 hour+ in duration Allow to wake naturally or wake after 1½ hours maximum Note: the window of wakefulness may extend to 3 hours, but don't extend unless your child no longer goes down easily within 2 hours and is also routinely sleeping through the night
Awake/leisure time Lunch	10–11.30 a.m.	Between the first and second nap, provide lunch with water The time will depend on wake time and nap duration There is a 3-hour window of wakefulness after Nap 1 ends and before Nap 2 needs to start Lunch should be over in time for the nap Follow your child's sleep cues or prepare for the nap 20 minutes before the end of the suggested waking period
Nap 2 – cot	11 a.m.–12.30 p.m.	Start time of Nap 2 depends on Nap 1 start time and duration Your child should be put down within 3 hours of waking from Nap 1

		Nap 2 will ideally be 1 hour+ in duration
		Allow to wake naturally or wake by 3.30 p.m. at the latest
Awake/leisure time Second feed and healthy snack	2–3 p.m.	Feed time/healthy snack time (depending on the previous feed) should happen after Nap 2
Possible nap as a back-up	3–4 p.m.	Your child may need a third nap between 3 and 4 p.m. if they haven't had enough sleep in the day. This can be a motion sleep
		Awake by 4.30 p.m. at the latest so that bedtime stays the same
		If naps have been short or finished too soon and you can't manage a third nap you may need to bring bedtime forward as far as 6 p.m. by adjusting the dinner and last feed and bringing the start of the bedtime routine forward by one hour
Dinner time	5–5.30 p.m.	Provide dinner – meat protein and carbohydrate
Final feed	6–6.15 p.m.	Provide bedtime feed
		Do this away from the bedroom, with the lights on, so that it has nothing to do with sleep
		Ensure a clear 45 minutes between end of feed and sleep time
Bedtime routine	6.20–6.30 p.m.	Start bath (if doing one) and/or the bedtime routine in the bedroom where your child will sleep
Into cot	6.50 p.m.	Place your child in the cot/use the stay-and-support approach as required
Aim to be asleep	7 p.m.	Aim for your child to be asleep, maintaining no more than a 4-hour window of wakefulness between the end of last nap and being in bed asleep
		If the final nap is finished early, bring bedtime forward to accommodate this

Twelve to eighteen months

Expectations

- Total amount of nighttime sleep: 10½–12 hours.
- Nighttime feeds are generally not required at this age and stage. If in doubt, discuss with your healthcare professional.
- Total amount of daytime sleep: 2¼–2½ hours.
- Number of naps: two.
- Milk need: 240–420ml twice per day and/or breastfeeds.
- Three solid meals/two to three healthy snacks/meat protein.

Daytime sleeping

I would anticipate a daytime sleep need in the region of two to two and a half hours, balanced between two naps. Most children under 16–18 months still benefit from a two-nap dynamic, especially if they do not routinely sleep through the night.

Some indicators of whether two naps are needed:

- If your child is not yet 18 months of age, does not sleep through the night and is tired by 10 a.m., two naps are needed.
- If your child can last until 11 a.m. it is possible that one nap is correct, but then that one nap needs to start closer to 12–12.30 p.m. in order to create the right balance. If this can be done either with immediate effect or gradually, moving the single nap by 15 minutes every two days, then follow the timetable for 18 months to two and a half years detailed below.
- If your child has a morning nap but then refuses the second nap, shorten the first nap to 45 minutes or one hour max and continue with two naps until the transition to one nap emerges properly (see Chapter 13).

Remember, even if you need to revisit two naps for a while, one nap is just around the corner!

A word about milk feeds

Your child's milk need has shrunk considerably now, to 230–400ml during the day. They should be eating three solid meals, two or three healthy snacks, as appropriate, and water throughout the day. If your child is drinking more than the suggested amounts a conscious effort to reduce would be advised and the sleep work may also help with this if there are still nighttime feeds!

Feeding and sleeping suggestions

Wake time First feed Breakfast	6–7.30 a.m.	From 6 a.m., and no later than 7.30 a.m., get up and start the day
		Provide first feed within the first half hour and breakfast within the next half hour
		Wake your child by 7.30 a.m. if still asleep to regulate body clock regardless of what has happened overnight
Nap 1 – cot	8–9.30 a.m.	This nap should start within 2–3 hours of waking
		Follow your child's sleep cues or prepare for this nap 20 minutes before the end of the suggested wake time
		This nap can be at least 45 minutes to 1 hour+ in duration
		Allow to wake naturally or wake after 1½ hours maximum – limit this further as outlined if necessary
		Note: the window of wakefulness may extend to 3 hours, but don't extend unless your child no longer goes down easily within 2 hours and is also routinely sleeping through the night

Awake/leisure time Lunch	10–11.30 a.m.	Between the first and second nap, provide lunch with water
		The time will depend on wake time and nap duration
		There is a 3-hour window of wakefulness after Nap 1 ends and before Nap 2 needs to start
		Lunch should be over in time for the nap
		Follow your child's sleep cues or prepare for the nap 20 minutes before the end of the suggested waking period
Nap 2 – cot	11 a.m.–12.30 p.m.	Start time of Nap 2 depends on Nap 1 start time and duration
		Your child should be put down within 3 hours of waking from Nap 1
		Pay attention to sleep signals
		Nap 2 will ideally be 1 hour+ in duration
		Allow to wake naturally or wake by 3.30 p.m. at the latest
Awake/leisure time Possible feed and healthy snack	3–3.30 p.m.	Feed time/healthy snack (depending on the previous feed) should happen after Nap 2
Possible nap as a back-up	3–4 p.m.	Your child may need a third nap between 3 and 4 p.m. if they haven't had enough sleep in the day. This can be a motion sleep
		Awake by 4.30 p.m. at the latest so that bedtime stays the same
		If naps have been short or finished too soon and you can't manage a third nap you may need to bring bedtime forward as far as 6 p.m. by adjusting the dinner and last feed and bringing the start of the bedtime routine forward by one hour

Dinner	5–5.30 p.m.	Provide dinner – meat protein and carbohydrate
Final feed	6–6.15 p.m.	Provide bedtime feed
		Do this away from the bedroom, with the lights on, so that it has nothing to do with sleep
		Ensure a clear 45 minutes between end of feed and sleep time
Bedtime routine	6.20–6.30 p.m.	Start bath (if doing one) and/or the bedtime routine in the bedroom where your child will sleep
Into cot	6.50 p.m.	Place your child in the cot/use the stay-and-support approach as required
Aim to be asleep	7 p.m.	Aim for your child to be asleep, maintaining no more than a 4-hour window of wakefulness between the end of last nap and being in bed asleep
		If the final nap is finished early, bring bedtime forward to accommodate this

Eighteen months to two and a half years

Expectations

- Total amount of nighttime sleep: 10½–12 hours.
- Nighttime feeds are generally not required at this age and stage. If in doubt, discuss with your healthcare professional.
- Total amount of daytime sleep: one to two hours+.
- Number of naps: one.
- Suggested milk need: 150ml per day and/or breastfeeds.
- Three solid meals/two to three healthy snacks/meat protein.

Your child's milk need is very low now, as little as 150ml, and this can be made up of dairy produce too. If you are still over-reliant on milk, start reducing – you will be surprised how milk can suppress a healthy daytime appetite.

Daytime sleeping

I would anticipate a daytime sleep need in the region of one to two hours, with most children in this age range able to manage on one nap per day.

If this is the case, this nap needs to start closer to 12.30–1 p.m. in order to create the right balance. If your child's current nap is earlier than this, judge the situation and think about gradually adjusting the single nap by 15 minutes every two days until the nap begins closer to 12.30–1 p.m. Don't be concerned with the wake period between getting up and the nap; it is the wake period between the nap and bedtime that has pernicious implications, if it's too long.

If your child is super tired by 10 a.m., provide a short cat nap of 30 minutes maximum and then a second main nap within three hours. You can do this until you feel your child is better rested.

Feeding and sleeping suggestions

Wake time First feed Breakfast	6–7.30 a.m.	From 6 a.m., and no later than 7.30 a.m., get up and start the day
		Provide first feed within the first half hour and breakfast within the next half hour
		Wake your child by 7.30 a.m. if still asleep to regulate body clock regardless of what has happened overnight
Awake/leisure time Lunch	11.30 a.m.– 12 p.m.	Have high-level activity in the morning and provide lunch with water
		Make sure lunch is done before the nap so that your child goes into the nap on a full stomach
Nap – cot	12.30–1 p.m.	Start of the single nap, ideally 1–2 hours+ in duration
		Allow to wake naturally or wake by 3.30 p.m. at the latest. If this nap starts to interfere with bedtime, wake at 3 p.m.
Possible drink and snack		Provide drink and healthy snack on waking

Dinner	5–5.30 p.m.	Provide dinner – meat protein and carbohydrate
Final feed	6–6.15 p.m.	Provide bedtime feed
		Do this away from the bedroom, with the lights on, so that it has nothing to do with sleep
		Ensure a clear 45 minutes between end of feed and sleep time
Bedtime routine	6.20–6.30 p.m.	Start bath (if doing one) and/or the bedtime routine in the bedroom where your child will sleep
Into cot	6.50 p.m.	Place your child in the cot/use the stay-and-support approach as required
Aim to be asleep at 7 p.m. to start with and adjust later as appropriate	7–8 p.m.	Aim for your child to be asleep, maintaining no more than a 4–5-hour window of wakefulness between the end of the nap and being in bed asleep
		If the nap is finished early, bring bedtime forward to accommodate this
		Aim for 7 p.m., but be prepared to adjust as your child gets better rested and a natural bedtime emerges – then prepare for bed 45 minutes before the bedtime that has become apparent

Two and a half to six years

Expectations

- Total amount of nighttime sleep: 10–13 hours.
- Nighttime feeds are generally not required at this age and stage. If in doubt, discuss with your healthcare professional.
- Total amount of daytime sleep: 0–2+ hours.
- Number of naps: none to one.
- Suggested milk need: 150ml per day and/or breastfeeds.
- Three solid meals/two to three healthy snacks/meat protein.

Your child's milk need is very low now, as little as 150ml, and this can be made up of dairy produce too. If you are still over-reliant on milk, start reducing – you will be surprised how milk can suppress a healthy daytime appetite.

Daytime sleeping

I would anticipate a daytime sleep need in the region of up to one and a half hours. Most children up to the age of three years are able to be on one nap per day. Beyond three years they will either reduce the length of their nap or will not need to nap every day as they work towards no nap somewhere between three and four years of age.

When they are napping, their single nap needs to start close to 12.30–1 p.m. in order to create the right balance. If their current nap is earlier than this, judge the situation and think about gradually adjusting the nap by 15 minutes every two days until the nap begins closer to 12.30–1 p.m. Don't be concerned with the wake period between getting up and the nap; it is the wake period between the nap and bedtime that has pernicious implications, if it's too long. Stop this nap around 3 p.m. initially and 2.30 p.m. if it starts to affect bedtime.

When your child is no longer napping, provide 'quiet time' for about an hour around the time when the nap used to happen, ideally reading, listening to music or audio books, but not watching television or electronic media.

Feeding and sleeping suggestions

Wake time Breakfast	6–7.30 a.m.	From 6 a.m., and no later than 7.30 a.m., get up and start the day
		Provide a drink within the first half hour and breakfast within the next half hour
		Wake your child by 7.30 a.m. if still asleep to regulate body clock regardless of what has happened overnight
Leisure time Lunch	11.30 a.m.– 12 p.m.	Have high-level activity in the morning time and provide lunch with water
		Make sure lunch is done before the nap (if applicable) so that your child goes into the nap on a full stomach

Nap or quiet time	12.30–1 p.m.	Start of the single nap, if needed, ideally 1–1½ hours in duration
		Allow to wake naturally or wake by 2.30–3 p.m. at the latest
		If this nap starts to interfere with bedtime, wake at 2.30 p.m.
		If no nap is required, encourage quiet time instead, around the same time frame as the nap – reading or listening to audio books, not television!
Leisure time Drink/snack		Provide drink and healthy snack on waking
		Ensure high-level activity in the afternoon
Dinner	5–5.30 p.m.	Provide dinner time – meat protein and carbohydrate
Final drinks	6.00–6.15pm	Provide bedtime drink/snack if applicable
		Do this away from the bedroom, with the lights on, so that it has nothing to do with sleep
Bedtime routine	6.20–6.30 p.m.	Start bath (if doing one) and/or the bedtime routine in the bedroom where your child will sleep
Into bed	6.50 p.m.	Have your child climb into bed/use the stay-and-support approach as required
Aim to be asleep at 7 p.m. initially and adjust later as appropriate	7–8.30 p.m.	Aim for your child to be asleep by 7 p.m., maintaining no more than a 4–5-hour window of wakefulness between the end of the nap and being in bed asleep
		If there is no nap, proceed as outlined and you can adjust as time moves on
		Aim for 7 p.m., but be prepared to adjust as your child gets better rested and a natural bedtime emerges. Then prepare for bed 45 minutes before this bedtime that has become apparent

Lucy Says

For many children now the day will be taken care of by preschool, Montessori, daycare and even big school. So the parts you can control will be in the evening. If your child has already started school it may be best to address the issues during the mid-term break or the holidays so that they are not even more overtired and trying to concentrate in school. You may also need to put on hold extracurricular activities – music, dancing, sport – that happen in the evening; just in the early stages of the process.

If you find that your child struggles to go to sleep much before 10 or 11 p.m. and then sleeps late in the morning, you will need to wake them early in the morning on the day you plan to start. In this case a nap may be needed, but this adjustment will help to establish bedtime and in turn a natural wake time.

Chapter 9

Developing the Daytime Routine

Now that you have reviewed the age-relevant feeding and sleeping suggestions, I want you to get a better understanding of why these recommendations and particular timings are effective and help you to avoid some typical errors that parents tend to make, and which can undermine the work you are doing. This chapter will deal with developing a daytime feeding and sleeping routine that is appropriate to you and your child.

Being informed

As your child develops, their sleep requirements also mature. Having an idea of how much sleep children need helps families have something to aim for. While individual children's specific sleep needs vary, there are general levels of most children's need for and timing of sleep.

Recommended daily sleep for children endorsed by the American Academy of Sleep Medicine as of 2016

Age	Amount of sleep required
4–12 months	12–16 hours*
1–2 years	11–14 hours*
3–5 years	10–13 hours*
6–12 years	9–12 hours
13–18 years	8–10 hours

Includes naps

Wake times

The basis of a good nighttime sleep starts first thing in the day. Not all wake times are equal. Our bodies are designed to start relatively early in the day. Waking between 6 a.m. and no later than 7.30 a.m. allows for the body to be hormone-regulated. Somehow, waking after 7.30 a.m., even by as little as 10 minutes, can have a disastrous impact on the rest of the day! Having a start time during this 6–7.30 a.m. bandwidth serves two main functions: it helps the body to establish the correct biological bedtime; and it also, in turn, helps to open up the natural times for your child's daytime sleep. So every adjustment that you will make is designed to have a positive impact on your child's overall sleeping pattern, and understanding that bedtime starts first thing in the day is a good start.

Lucy Says

Starting the day between 6 a.m. and no later than 7.30 a.m., although difficult when you are tired, has an immediate positive impact on sleeping patterns and should be observed with regularity.

Here are some common mistakes around wake time.

- Your child is awake at any time from 6 a.m., but you don't get up until 7 a.m. or later; instead you hang around the bed or bedroom, and you might even do the morning feed before leaving the room. I recommend that you get up and start the day if your child wakes in this time frame. Get up, leave the room, have the morning feed outside the bedroom – separate from sleep. Expose your child to light to help reset the body clock and use lighting to regulate sleeping patterns.

- Your child is awake a lot overnight so when they are asleep in the morning parents are reluctant to wake them. This is a fundamental sleep mistake. Waking by 7.30 a.m. is a must if you want to stop perpetuating the sleep difficulties that you have. So create a new rule – you will wake your child by 7.30 a.m., regardless of what has happened overnight.

- Your child is awake at an appropriate time, but you don't provide their feed or their breakfast until later. Very often parents will tell me that their child is awake at 6 a.m. but they don't feed them until 7 a.m. I understand that parents are reluctant to condition their child to have a feed before a certain time that the parents have earmarked, but if you don't feed within 30 minutes of awakening you potentially deregulate the day from a feeding and sleeping perspective. My general recommendation is to feed your child their milk, breast or bottle within 30 minutes of waking and eat breakfast, when established, in the next half hour too. Delaying breakfast has the same effect, and if your child is under 12 months, your delayed breakfast may interfere with your first nap. Even if your child is going to childcare and will be having breakfast there, I believe that they should have something to eat within the first hour of waking.

- Your child is awake at an appropriate time but they are not interested in their morning feed due to a nighttime feed. It is very important to establish and maintain your morning feed. Generally, this resistance to eat may indicate that the night feed is not necessary anymore (more on nighttime feeds to come). When you see this presentation you need to focus on re-establishing the morning feed on wake up, by either age appropriately night weaning or at least reducing so that the morning feed can start the day feeds off for you. As you begin, offer the feed anyway, even if your child is not really interested and has fed not that long ago overnight. Provide the feed and count it as your first feed so that you can run the feed timings throughout the rest of the day and are not always playing catch up. If you are night weaning then re-establishing this feed will be simple, you just need to allow for it.

Daytime sleep issues

Daytime sleep has a large controlling impact on your child's ability to sleep well overnight. The dynamic between *each* daytime sleep is also important. Limiting your child's daytime sleep to improve nighttime sleep *may* sometimes work to your advantage, but in my experience, it may only improve the nighttime presentation in the short term and then the issues re-emerge within 10–14 days, sometimes worse than they were originally. Or you may be confused as your child naps incredibly well during the day and still you have sleep issues overnight.

Here are some common nap issues.

1. Your child takes inadequate daytime sleep, may be easy or difficult to put down in the cot or the buggy or car, but the nap never exceeds 45 minutes. Although they may have a series of short naps, this may not be enough to meet your child's sleep need, resulting in an overtired child at bedtime who will either be challenging to get to sleep or easy, but will wake frequently throughout the course of the night and maybe even stay awake for large periods of time during the core part of the night.

2. Your child may take excellent daytime sleep, but the balance may not be right. When I refer to balance it is because each nap

takes the sleep pressure off the brain, but certain times during the day are more significant than others. One of the most pernicious nap dynamics is what I call a 'top-heavy' day. This involves your child taking a marathon first nap in the morning, for one or two hours or more, and then weaker or no more sleep for the rest of the day. This creates too long a wakeful period before bedtime, which in turn enables frustrating sleep problems. Whether your child requires one, two or four naps in the day (according to age), the first two naps are the most significant. However, you may need to be aware of what I call the 'power play' between Nap 1 and Nap 2. Bear in mind that you will retain the first two daytime sleeps until your child is closer to 15–18 months of age, *but the second nap is the more significant.* There is a very real competition between these two sleeps, with Nap 1 wanting to be stronger and longer and Nap 2, as a result, being weaker (less than one hour). The ideal is that Naps 1 and 2 are of equal or similar duration, and this comes down to your child. If only one nap is over one hour, you need it to be Nap 2. Nap 2 carries the weight until bedtime, so that your child is not overtired at the onset of bedtime and is able to go to sleep. Keep this dynamic in mind when we start to address the age-appropriate timetable for your child.

3. You may find that no matter how early you prepare for a nap, how well you read sleep signals, the nap is still hard to achieve and even harder to maintain. This can be caused by too late a bedtime and/or frequent awakenings through the night, resulting in an under-rested child before the day has even started. This feeds the cycle of tiredness and perpetuates the problem. By beginning to implement the age-related feeding and sleeping balances suggested for your child, you will help to unlock your child's mechanism for both nighttime and daytime sleep – this will take time but slight improvements may be seen from the start.

4. If your child is dependent in the context of their bedtime sleep (uses a bottle/rocking/nursing/requires a parent), that alone

can make naps hard to land. Even with the most accurate timing your child may struggle to achieve and maintain their naps, so the answer is to start to work on all your child's sleep issues, aiming to strengthen their biological timekeeping and weakening the dependencies, using my stay-and-support approach.

Bedtimes

One of the main causes of many childhood sleep issues may be a bedtime that is attempted too late. This is the foundation of a lot the problems experienced by parents. With children older than six months up to age six, bedtime generally needs to be somewhere between 6 p.m. and 8 p.m. All children are different, but they are biologically programmed to get tired and be 'sleep ready' in this time frame.

Many families I work with have a bedtime that is outside this recommended bandwidth and so it will need to be adjusted significantly as we correct the issues. That is not to say that you will always have to operate an early bedtime, but it will definitely be the basis of any sleep strategy that I put together, for two main reasons: your child's body will be getting ready for sleep in this time frame; and their brain will be open to learning a 'new' way of going to sleep; this strategy on its own is part of the successful formula that I apply.

Lucy Says

If you attempt to correct sleep issues without setting the right bedtime, you may well be successful, but on the other hand you may not, and you may find your child is extremely upset and just not able to gain the skill that you are trying to establish.

The early bedtime

Bringing forward bedtime, just like having a regular wake time, helps to first of all *make the learning process easier for your child*, but the earlier onset of sleep also helps to unlock the daytime sleeping mechanism too. Many parents will be concerned that an early bedtime may result in their child waking at 4 a.m. to start the day, or they may report that they tried an early bedtime before and the child woke earlier or more frequently than ever before. First of all, the early bedtime will not mean your child will start the day too early; in fact the opposite is true. Of course the wake time may get earlier, but it will also be in conjunction with sleeping through the night and on that basis, beyond 6 a.m. is reasonable – provided they have had enough hours and they have consolidated their nighttime sleep. Furthermore, at the very start of your sleep plan you may experience early waking, but that will pass as positive sleeping habits become more established.

Bedtime concerns

If you have attempted an earlier bedtime before only for it to backfire and produce more frequent waking or your child appeared to treat it as a nap, that may be due to many reasons. The brain may need to process the change and as a result the child wakes frequently in the short term, but if you continue and you put together all the recommendations – both timetable and strategy – uninterrupted sleep is coming your way. It is not unusual for a plan for sleep, once implemented, to make everything worse at the start – that is a very normal presentation – but as quickly as it regresses, sleep regroups and it will start to get better and everyone can get the sleep that they need.

Lucy Says

Any changes may result in your child's sleep getting worse before it gets better, but with patience and commitment it will improve.

Many families, on the other hand, *are* operating what appears to be an appropriate bedtime (in the region of 6–8 p.m.), but due to the nature of their ongoing issues, *even that time is too late*. So it would not be unusual for me to explain that even 7.30 p.m. is too late for their child while they are having issues, and that we need to prepare for bed earlier as a result.

Furthermore, a common misconception can arise between the time you *commence* your child's sleep process and the time they actually go to sleep. Many parents tell me that bedtime is 7.30 p.m., but this is only the time that they begin the process and their child is not asleep until 8.15 p.m.

Lucy Says

To help promote better sleep you will need:

- A regular wake time, no later than 7.30 a.m.
- Adequate age-relevant daytime sleep
- An age-appropriate bedtime.

You will be aware now that having regularity in your day and creating a feeding and sleeping balance for your child is crucial to the success of your sleep plan.

Now I want to walk you through the age-relevant sleeping and feeding suggestions for your child, taking note of the important elements outlined below.

Daytime feeding and sleeping suggestions

The feeding and sleeping suggestions provided in Chapters 7 and 8 are the 'gold standard'. In other words this is where we are heading. It won't look like the ideal to start with – it may never entirely match – but we need something to aim for. This what we are *trying* to achieve. I will give you some landmarks and guidelines to help you make progress.

At the conclusion of your sleep learning exercise, you will be able to have a bedtime routine, place your baby in their cot, say goodnight and walk away and they will be able to put themselves to sleep with minimised parental input at bedtime and overnight. This is our goal, but we have a lot of work to do first and this is our starting point. You are likely three to four weeks away from your sleep lottery win.

You will need to ensure that your child is getting enough to eat and drink throughout the course of the day. My feeding and sleeping suggestions outline some feeding amounts by age, but always ask your healthcare professional if unsure. Your child also needs to be getting food at the right time, so remember how much emphasis I place on the evening meal. In tandem with this, the digestive tract should be relaxed in advance of sleep, so I advise a minimum window of two hours between the last meal and being in bed asleep.

Many parents whose children are drinking excessive quantities of milk during the night will report that they show a lack of interest in either eating or drinking during the day. Once you have established with your doctor your particular child's nighttime feed need, if any, a night weaning process – outlined in Chapter 10 – will help the daytime appetite improve. This may take three to seven days to settle in, and often there's a void, when your child does not immediately start eating better, but be patient – it will come. Furthermore, a peripheral positive knock-on effect is that most parents who complete the sleep learning process observe better appetites and a greater willingness to try new food.

Lucy Says

As you night wean it can take three to seven days for the day appetite to emerge – and it will.

Waking and breakfast guide

In order to break the cycle of waking and feeding and even bed-sharing, from night one onwards we are going to treat any waking before 6 a.m. as nighttime waking and we are going to apply the consistent stay-and-support approach that you are now familiar with.

Beyond 6 a.m., if your child is awake, bright-eyed and ready to go, I would never try to extend the night by sleep learning, feeding or bed-sharing. Just press start on the day, get up and begin the breakfast routine. Obviously if your child wakes around this time and is groggy and appears open to going back to sleep, then of course try to extend the night, but not if they are awake and looking to get up.

Lucy Says

Don't start the day any later than 7.30 a.m., regardless of what has happened overnight.

On the flip side, if your child is still asleep, even if you have had a horrible or tough night, even if they have stayed awake for a long time and only gone back to sleep around 5 a.m., wake them no later than 7.30 a.m. If your child is habitually awake from 5 a.m. onwards, this may not be part of your vocabulary, but I just want you to know how to respond to every eventuality. So, by 7.30 you're up and about and ready to sort breakfast.

I would advise that your child has their morning feed within 30 minutes of getting up and eats their breakfast within 30 minutes of the feed. This can happen in reverse order, provided there is no resistance to either. Basically, your child will have their milk and breakfast (when applicable) within the first hour of waking; this regulates their blood sugar levels, anchors your day for feeding and also helps you to be able to prepare for the first nap in a timely fashion.

The first nap

Follow the recommended suggested wake period that is relevant to your child's age. I anticipate that your child will need to be prepared for the first nap of the day within two to three hours after breakfast, depending on their age. Notice that I say *within* two to three hours. If the suggested wakeful period for your child's age category is two hours, you need to aim for your child to be asleep *within* this time frame. So I advise that you follow their lead – as in the sleep cues we discussed – or the time on the clock, whichever comes first. If you don't see a sleep cue, and this could be for a variety of reasons (they're good at hiding, you miss the cue, you're dealing with an older sibling), I would always prepare for that nap within *20 minutes before the end* of your suggested wakeful period. This may sound a bit prescriptive, but it gives you a chance to have something to work on – if you don't see the signs. Over time, this will become part of how you operate and the fabric of your lifestyle, but as you work on the issues, it gives you a place to start.

Lucy Says

If at first you find it hard to read sleep cues, prepare for the nap 20 minutes before the end of the maximum suggested wake time.

That first nap can be as short as 40–45 minutes; it may be as long as an hour plus in duration. The duration will ultimately come down to your own child's sleep need. I would advise that you allow your child to wake naturally, but I would wake them after an hour and a half (this may not be part of your vocabulary either but we'll aim high!). If your child is 12 months plus, you may need to wake them after one hour to create enough space for Nap 2.

Lucy Says

If the second nap is hard to achieve, wake your child from Nap 1 after a maximum of one and a half hours if under 12 months and one hour if over 12 months.

Ideally, once you have begun, you will aim for the first and second sleep to be in a cot in a sleep environment.

When your child has had their first nap, whatever the length (we can discuss extending naps later on), you will organise the suggested wakeful period before the second nap of the day.

Between the end of Nap 1 and the start of Nap 2, there will be a wakeful period of two to three hours, depending on which age-relevant timetable you are observing. Once again, I want you to follow the child's lead, or the time on the clock, whichever comes first; and prepare 20 minutes before the end of this wakeful period, in the absence of a sleep cue. Many parents will report that within 45 minutes of being awake their child is yawning, but I recommend that you ignore this and allow at least an hour and a half to pass before attempting another daytime sleep as the sleep drive will not be strong enough for your child to go to sleep easily.

Lucy Says

If your child has already had one nap today (even if short), ignore sleep cues before an hour and a half has passed and don't prepare for another nap until then.

Between the first and second nap I suggest that you provide their second milk (if under eight months) of the day and lunch, if you have started on solid foods. Lunch with young children is generally early – mid-morning – it is not lunchtime as we think of it. It may seem unrealistic to us as adults, but is appropriate for a young child and is helping you create the feeding and sleeping balance that is required. So, provide the second milk feed if still appropriate and lunch. This needs to happen before the second sleep so that they go into this sleep on a full stomach and they're not woken by hunger. If your child is eight months plus, the mid-morning milk feed is normally dropped in preference to the introduction of meat protein. So lunch from eight months onwards is taken with a drink of water.

Lucy Says

If your child is eight months plus and you are still giving a mid-morning milk feed and overnight feeds, eliminate the overnight feeds first before you drop this bottle.

The second nap

This second sleep will ideally be an hour plus in duration. This won't necessarily happen to start with, but this is where we are heading. We will be making every effort to help extend and promote *this sleep* so that it can carry the weight of the day – more to follow in our chapter on naps.

Allow your child to wake naturally and only wake them if they look likely to sleep through their next milk feed, which will be due around 2–3 p.m., depending on your other feed times. This may not be relevant to begin with, but keep it in mind as you progress.

After the second sleep, it is a good idea to have another milk feed (for children up to 12 months plus) and a suitable healthy snack.

Lucy Says

Your child will need Nap 1 and Nap 2 until they get to around 16–18 months of age.

The third nap (under eight months)

This nap is still very important and generally needs to happen within one and a half and two and a half hours of the end of Nap 2. Again, observe your child's body language and provide for this nap accordingly. Although this nap is crucial and helps balance the day until bedtime, it actually doesn't matter where it happens – I suggest that you *don't* use the cot for this nap but think of it as an 'any way that works' nap. For example, use the buggy (either in the house or on a walk), the swing, the car, the sling. If you are trying to weaken an arms/feeding or bed-sharing dependency, it may be best to avoid your old habits and work on relocating Nap 3.

This nap can be as little as 10 minutes *or* as much as an hour plus in duration. The length is not that relevant, but it needs to be over by 4.30/5 p.m. at the latest. Don't be afraid of napping close to 5 p.m. – but not after – that is the perfect dynamic to arrive comfortably at a 7 p.m. bedtime. Most babies benefit from a wake period of about two hours between the final nap and being in bed asleep, until they are better rested.

Lucy Says

Nap 3 can be hard to achieve and will be gone by eight months plus, so don't use the cot – use the car or the buggy instead.

If your child is eight months or older and if naps have been short or are top-heavy in the day, you may well need to do a third sleep as a filler. This can also can happen in the car or buggy and needs to be finished by 4.30 p.m. at the latest. This is temporary – just while you help establish daytime sleep. What you really need to be mindful of is that initially your child should not be awake for more than four hours between the end of the Nap 2 and bedtime. This may extend to five hours when your child is 18 months plus and, of course, sleeping through the night.

Lucy Says

Use an additional nap if the day is short on sleep or naps are finished too early in the day.

Closing the gap

If the gap between the final nap and bedtime is longer than advised in your age-relevant timetable, either operate Nap 3 or, if this means that your day is finishing too early for naps or you can't manage another nap, then bring forward bedtime to 6 p.m. onwards. Please don't be afraid of the super early bedtime; it is not a long-term solution, but it can be a great short-term solution as you work through the process to prevent an overtired and sleep-resistant child at bedtime, which is our key learning opportunity.

Lucy Says

If naps are finished early in the day and you can't manage a third nap, aim for an early bedtime of 6 p.m. onwards. Don't be afraid of this!

Dinner and bedtime milk feed

Dinner would ideally be at around 5–5.30 p.m. once solid food is established, or as early as you can make it, based on collecting the child and coming home from work, if applicable. I strongly recommend that this is an evening meal-type food – a meat protein (once age-appropriate and established in the diet) and carbohydrate-based meal. Very often young children have a dinner at lunchtime and a lighter food in the evening and I would either swap that around or have two dinner-type meals. Between dinner and morning time is the longest time that you require your child to fast, so it will need to be sustaining and offer a slow energy release. You are not trying to stack up the calories ahead of sleep – this will

143

rarely work anyway – and you are in no way trying to drop a night feed if this is still relevant, but it is a good idea to ensure that your child, even if they're not hungry, does not wake because they don't feel full.

Lucy Says

Once dinner is over I suggest you provide your last feed at around 6–6.15 p.m. I like this to be entirely separate from sleep to weaken any feeding associations and to observe good dental hygiene, with an opportunity to brush teeth (when they have erupted) before sleep.

I recommend that this feed is done in the living space, with the lights on and with your child in their day clothes, so that there's nothing to do with sleep. I encourage you to consider a drink before bedtime, whether breast or bottle, and I discourage you to use this as a relaxant to help wind your child down. Although I am aware that this *can* relax them, I also see hundreds of families using this practice to achieve sleep when it's actually part of the sleep problem in the first place. Creating clearance of at least 45 minutes between the end of the feed and being in bed and asleep is a good yardstick and helps us to be sure that the feed is not even *partially* helping sleep happen – which can in turn contribute to frequent night waking or long wake periods and/or early rising. Finally, if you are worried that your child is not drinking enough, first review their daily intake and be aware that the amount taken throughout the day is more significant than what happens in the last hour before bedtime. If you are super concerned and your child won't take the feed, then you could have the feed in the bedroom with the lights on at the start of the bedtime routine, but this is not my preference as it can still be part of helping induce sleep or, indeed, cause a micro sleep that recharges the batteries and makes it increasingly difficult for your child to go to sleep.

Lucy Says

Make sure milk feeds are finished 45 minutes before bedtime.

The bedtime routine

Finally, I suggest that you prepare for your bedtime routine at around 6.20–6.30 p.m. to begin with. I know that this can put many working parents under pressure, so start the process going into a weekend so that you are not rushing. It won't be fixed within a weekend, but it helps to get you off on the right foot and then as better sleep is evolving you can start the process slightly later. Don't forget that a bedtime that's too late contributes to many of the sleep problems that parents experience and very often this subtle adjustment can help your child go to sleep more easily and in turn stay asleep for as long as their body requires.

So start the bedtime process at around 6.20–6.30 p.m. If you are committed to a bath, I would do this now, after the feed. I have to mention that I am not always in favour of a bath before bedtime. Of course I understand the principle that it can help relax a child, but the main premise of it is to help the body temperature drop and help sleep that way – as well as being a cue. If you are operating my wakeful suggestions, the body temperature will be dropping anyway and the bedtime routine is recognisable enough for your child to understand.

I also think that a bath at this time is a big job, especially for working parents, and I often save a bath for non-sleep time and treat it like an activity. You will decide what you can commit to and of course it doesn't need to be every night if you do. For me what is important is the bedtime routine, so I suggest that you feed in the living space, then bath (if you decide to do it) and obviously teeth/wash up if you don't, then the bedtime routine in your child's bedroom.

145

- If there is no bath – feed and then bedtime routine.
- If there is a bath – feed, bath, bedtime routine. Spend no more than 45 minutes on the entire process.

In the absence of the bath I suggest a 20–30-minute wind-down, in the bedroom where your child will sleep. Don't operate a bedtime routine that is 'fractured' between the living room and your bedroom. Everything to do with their sleep should happen in the child's bedroom (with the exception of teeth clean/wash/bath).

Starting the new routine

You will need to pay careful attention to the (perhaps new) wake and sleep times. If you feel, once you have reviewed the timetables, that your original routine and mine are radically different or if for some reason, like vaccinations or a break away, you are not starting the process immediately, you could choose to do what I call 'timetabling' for a few days or more.

This involves *making no changes except for the timings*. If you typically feed, nurse or rock your baby at sleep times, then continue to do this but operate my timing suggestions. This won't necessarily make a huge difference, but sometimes it can. More important, it will potentially help programme your child for better sleep as you move on. Many families describe this period as a mixed bag. Either way, you will begin soon and when you do, it will be a two-pronged approach, using both the timings and my stay-and-support approach for better sleep.

Lucy Says

Before you begin the sleep learning exercise you could spend three to seven days or more making no other changes except the timetable.

Chapter 10

The Overnight Plan

I f you are phasing out rocking, bed-sharing/swapping, buggy or dummy use, for example, when your child wakes during the night, respond quickly by going to them. Later on you can delay going to them immediately, but at the start of this process, if your child wakes overnight, go quickly to the bedroom where they are sleeping and repeat the stay-and-support approach. Use the new style of support for your child each and every time they wake.

If your child is in their own bed and can wander into your bedroom, meet them as soon as you can, limit talk and touching and 'herd' them back into bed, getting them to climb back into the bed themselves and pull the covers up themselves. Don't lift them or allow hand-holding so that you don't encourage the waking. Your child needs to learn how to sleep independently, and this is the beginning of the process.

Lucy Says

If you are transitioning from holding, rocking, rolling, bed-sharing/swapping or dropping the dummy, then return to the bedroom – if you have kept the dummy, do a dummy run and leave; if you have dropped the dummy or if you don't have a dummy to start with, return to the cot or bedside and use the stay-and-support approach each and every time your child wakes, until at least 6 a.m., then get up and start the day.

This can of course be the challenging part and as the night unfolds it is possible that your child could stay awake for an extended period of time as you weaken their expectation of being rocked or brought into your or the spare bed. It can be usual for this element to take one to two hours at the start. They might not cry or be upset and protesting all this time, but they might just find it hard – as will you. You might be inclined to bring them into the bed, or rock them back to sleep, because you know that this works, but you must also acknowledge that this is just a crisis management approach and will not help your child to learn to cycle through those nighttime sleep phases. So although you will be tired and you may not get much sleep, this bit gets easier quickly and then you know there will be an end to your sleep struggles. Some parents report multiple quick wakings, some extended wake periods and some multiple waking and returning to sleep only to wake again. Families ask me 'Is it normal?', and I would suggest that this is *your* normal and *your* journey and it most certainly will start to improve. Most families report that by night 10–14 they have had some consolidated nights. The older child may take closer to 21 nights before you start to see any progress.

If you are not progressing beyond this time frame, it may indicate that something is not currently being implemented as well as your child requires – this can be anything from a nap imbalance, overtiredness at bedtime or one or two nights when you didn't always see through the sleep learning exercise. Every decision that you make overnight has a direct effect on the success of your plan and operating with precision and deviating from the suggestions will start to confuse your child and may also cause much more upset than anyone wants – and, of course, still not get the result you want.

So be patient and calm; it takes time for anyone to learn something new.

Nighttime feeds

If you have been using feeds as a means to return your child to sleep you will have to review your night feed approach and factor in some changes.

One of the most typical issues overnight is the feed, whether breast or bottle, to help your child go back to sleep.

First, consider whether your child *needs* a nighttime feed? Try not to base the answer on the fact that they drink it so that *must* mean they need it. Not necessarily. Obviously this decision will need to be age-appropriate. I generally suggest that under six to seven months, most children may need a nighttime feed, but beyond that age, once solids are established and meat protein is in the diet, the reason for feeding can start to be more than hunger. If you are stuck in a regular nighttime feed scenario, your child may need the feed not for nutritional reasons but because of association; feeding and sleeping have become interlinked and hunger has become conditioned.

Frequent nighttime feeders can often drink more than their daily requirement of milk intake in the overnight period alone. Biologically unnecessary feeds wake up the digestive system when it should be sleeping, cause overfull nappies, and may increase the risk of dental decay. Furthermore, it will absolutely compromise their daytime appetite for both solid food and milk. Over-reliance on milk when your child is beyond 12 months (also very common) may start to cause an iron deficiency issue – over-consumption of milk prevents iron absorption. Iron deficiency can also contribute to sleep difficulties.

Beyond six to seven months of age, and generally by nine months, there is little evidence to suggest that typically developing children require nighttime feeds. Of course there will be exceptions to this but if in doubt, keep a food diary and seek advice from your GP or health visitor; they can assess what you are doing, weigh your child and confirm whether night feeds are still required and you can allow for that accordingly. If you do have an older child who still requires a night feed, it will normally be only one feed, not a series of feeds.

Lucy Says

Some parents keep providing night bottles because the day appetite is not adequate. This is, of course, part of the reason for the diminished day appetite and would be a disservice to the child if not addressed. Beyond nine months solid food intake begins to take over from milk, but if the milk is still offered in large quantities this relationship doesn't get a chance to evolve.

As your child heads towards 12 months of age the milk is not a nutritional powerhouse and it won't keep them feeling full anyway – that time has passed. Furthermore, it is the brain that needs to sleep and the stomach will follow. Obviously, if your child is hungry they may not sleep well, but many children in my practice eat and drink more than the recommended amounts and *still* don't sleep – it is not a hunger problem but a sleep association one.

Typically the issue of excessive nighttime feeds is caused by the dependency on feeds at bedtime or an historic dependency either at bedtime or filtered into overnight. If your child can only get to sleep by sucking a bottle of milk or the breast, or the feed is the last thing you do before bedtime, then, as your child cycles through sleep, they may need to have a feed to allow this to happen. Children will wake frequently overnight for a milk feed when the feeding plays a significant role in bedtime, either currently or historically. It will become a feeding and sleeping association and a potentially conditioned hunger rather than hunger itself.

I encourage parents to work on separating out the feed from sleep. Provide the feed in the living space, as outlined, before you begin the bedtime wind-down or bath, so that the feed is at the *very start* of the bedtime routine. When you make this change you may find that your child struggles to go to sleep without the aid of the feed. This indicates their reliance on the feed to achieve a sleepy state, and then you will need to implement my stay-and-support approach.

Lucy Says

Be aware that your child doesn't always have to go all the way to sleep on the feed. Sometimes the feed can be just too close to sleep time and, although your child appears awake, a sleepy state has been induced by the feeding act. As a result they wake frequently all night long.

To make sure this doesn't happen, I strongly reiterate that the last feed should be provided *at least* 45 minutes before sleep time and ideally *not* in the bedroom. This way, your child can have their drink and then brush their teeth, when applicable, before the bedtime routine.

Another typical scenario is a child who can put themselves to sleep without a feed or any other intervention, but still requires night feeds. These wakings may initially have stemmed from nap deprivation or a late bedtime and are quickly transformed into a conditioned hunger from regular milk intake overnight. Of course, if you yourself were habitually fed during the nighttime, then over time you would begin to feel hungry around this time and start to need this meal.

The ultimate aim, once you have the consent from your GP or health visitor, is to eliminate the night feeds so that your child can sleep through the night with reduced parental input and you can help improve and enhance the daytime appetite for food and milk.

There are many options for parents hoping to wean night bottles, ranging from cold turkey to diluting, dream feeding or reducing. My recommendation would be a regulated and reducing approach over the course of a number of nights, provided all the other measures are in place.

Each baby is different, but here are some common types of night feeds which may help you identify your situation. Which category are you in?

- ☑ The drip feed: Often parents report that they use one bottle over the course of the night with the child taking sups at each waking, or that the breastfed baby feeds frequently throughout the night, not staying on the breast for very long.

- ☑ The big feed: Sometimes the child wakes and drinks a full bottle or one or both breasts on each awakening.

- ☑ The unmanaged dream feed: Other parents use a 'dream feed' or 'sleepy feed'. They wake their child at a certain point in the night, generally before the parents' bedtime, on the premise that they will then sleep until the morning. Obviously this can be effective and it does suit many children, but it can also be very unsuitable, resulting in a dream feed at the start of the night and a succession of wakes to feed thereafter, signalling that the dream feed concept in this case does not suit your child.

Lucy Says

Some children drip feed through the night.

Others drink full amounts each time they wake.

Some have a dream feed or sleepy feed and sleep until morning.

Others have a dream feed or sleepy feed and wake multiple times for more feeds thereafter.

It is not easy to break any of these cycles and as you do, ensure that you offer extra ounces or increased breastfeeds and solid food as the days unfold, even if this means not entirely following the daytime feeding suggestions in your age-relevant time structure – this will emerge as time goes by.

It may take three to seven days for a daytime appetite to manifest itself and improve, and it can also take 10 nights plus for night waking to disappear. As long as you feel that you are making improvements incrementally, you should persevere. If no progress is being made – the child is still waking frequently or taking ages to resettle – maybe other elements are not correctly in place and you will need to review the situation. More on this as we move through the stages and troubleshoot (see Chapter 13).

Lucy Says

When making changes towards positive sleep habits parents typically report their child's increased appetite, enhanced mood and behaviour and longer stretches of sleep between wake-ups. If this is happening then keep going, you are on the right track!

Weakening the feeding cycle

Here is a night-weaning approach for your bottle or breastfed baby. First you should check with your health professional that it is appropriate for your child. You should also implement my daytime feeding and sleeping suggestions and begin the sleep learning stay-and-support approach at bedtime.

Regulating multiple feeds

I recommend that parents regulate the number of feeds and at the same time reduce the intake so that within only four nights there are no night feeds and plenty of learning opportunities to return to sleep without suckling. And, of course, the child's body is getting less used to the calories. Typically, once all the other sleep suggestions are being correctly applied, within seven nights (or less) of no overnight feed you will experience your first almost or complete sleep through the night!

If you feed on multiple occasions or use more than one bottle or breastfeed to maintain your child's sleep, this is how to regulate the nighttime feeds:

- Decide on night one of the process to provide two feeds overnight within four hours of each other. If it is a bottle, prepare two bottles containing your usual amount (normally between 150ml and 240ml – for breastfeeds it's usually five minutes to 20 minutes, in my experience).

Lucy Says

Some feeding times on the breast are much longer, mostly driven by comfort, so then I suggest actively unlatching after the first 10 minutes or so of sucking and swallowing as you begin.

- Decide that your child must go four hours between the initial bedtime feed and the first night feed. This means that if your child's last feed is at around 6 p.m. they will not be due a feed before 10 p.m.
- If your child wakes before four hours/10 p.m., use the stay-and-support sleep learning approach detailed in Chapter 5 and already implemented at bedtime.

Lucy Says

You don't need to wake your baby after 4 hours; wait for them to wake naturally, even if you have been using a dream or sleepy feed.

- On first wake after four hours or more after the bedtime feed, you can provide a breastfeed or bottle. Allow them to drink as much as they like and they may return to sleep on this. Actively unlatch after sucking and swallowing as appropriate. Return to the cot and start the four-hour window again.
- If your child wakes before four hours after the first nighttime feed, use the stay-and-support approach.
- If they wake after another four plus hours, provide the second feed. Once again allow them to drink as much as they want. They may return to sleep on this.
- For any waking after the second nighttime feed and before 6 a.m., implement the stay-and-support approach.
- Remember that any waking before 6 a.m. is a night waking and needs to be treated as such.
- After 6 a.m., if your child is awake or has stayed awake from an earlier hour, do an exaggerated wake-up and start the day.
- Go downstairs and begin breakfast, avoiding your bed or bedroom.

Lucy Says

The exaggerated wake-up means leaving the room for a moment so that you change the dynamic and avoid teaching your child to cry or wait for you to give in. Return to the bedroom, big rise and shine, open curtains, turn on the lights, get up and start the day.

Night-weaning multiple feeds

Once you begin to regulate the night feeds, immediately begin to reduce them as well.

- Over three nights, reduce the amount in the bottle or the time on the breast by one-third so that you are providing about 60–90ml or two to four minutes by night three. For example:

	Bottle	Breast
Night 1	210ml	10 minutes (actively unlatch if necessary)
Night 2	120ml	6 minutes
Night 3	60ml	3 minutes
Night 4	No feeds	

- Continue to run the four-hour concept (see above) and use the stay-and-support approach if your child does not return to sleep on the reduced amount.
- It may be far easier for the breastfed baby to be resettled by the parent who is not breastfeeding and for mum to just appear for the feed.
- If mum has to do the settling, wear a high-neck, long-sleeved, newly laundered top – or the other parent's top if it will fit!
- On the fourth night you will not provide a nighttime feed. You will use the stay-and-support approach all night from bedtime until 6 a.m. at the earliest.
- Resist the urge to introduce a water bottle as this may

just become a replacement. If thirst is a concern consider a sippy cup of water, but beware – this may also become a replacement.

- Nights four and five are usually challenging for both parent and child, but stay positive: by day 11 of starting the process, so after a week of no feeds, you will likely be starting to see a massive improvement.

Lucy Says

Some parents feel overwhelmed by the speed of the weaning process. You can go more slowly, but I feel you prolong the agony for the child and delay your results and you may run out of steam. The idea is to reduce the body's calorie intake and then help your child become more efficient with their own sleep process. This *is* an effective approach.

Night-weaning a single feed

If historically there is only one nighttime feed, fed all in one go, you don't need to do the two-feeds approach. You just need to decide *when* that single feed should happen. You've seen that I consider anything before 6 a.m. as nighttime, so even if the single night feed happens in the early hours of the morning, although *you* may consider it to be the first feed of the day, if it happens before 6 a.m. or, indeed, if it is provided to extend nighttime sleep, it is still a night feed and will be viewed as such by your child's brain.

Many families describe their weaning process as retaining a feed at 5 a.m., only to discover that gradually the child begins to wake earlier and earlier until they are back to where they were at the beginning, or very close to it.

Simply put, if your child no longer needs a nighttime feed as per their age and stage, there should be no feeds until morning and they should be provided separately from sleep. Doing it any other way can undermine the sleep work.

Lucy Says

I know that a great many parents enjoy cuddles and feeds in the big bed first thing in the morning, but this may need to be put on hold until the expectations around night activity are dissolved. Otherwise you are in danger of giving mixed messages, which means that you may not reach your goals. So put on hold and revisit at a later date.

Does your child still need a night feed?

If you and your GP still feel that your child needs a night feed and this is an informed decision – not just based on the fact that they always drink a bottle or because they fail to eat or drink much during the day – you can work with this and retain one or two night feeds. Understand that sometimes if you retain biologically unnecessary feeds, this stops the nights consolidating and can in turn stop the naps from improving too.

When this is relevant, I would first use the regulating approach as outlined above for either one or two night feeds and ignore the weaning process for one or both of the feeds, as required. If you proceed on this basis and within 10–14 days your child is still waking on extra occasions between feeds for more than a dummy re-plug, it may indicate that they just 'don't get it' – why they can be fed sometimes and not at other times. If this is the case, I would introduce a fixed feed approach in which you initiate the feed (whether it is one feed or two). Set an alarm, lift your child from their sleep and provide a night feed, and every other time they wake, just resettle them. This method helps you see if they can sleep for a longer time without a feed. In some cases one or both feeds can be dropped, but it also allows for a feed for as long as you deem appropriate without causing mixed messages in the long term. In time, if you start to feel that the feed or feeds are no longer required, you can reduce the contents in the bottle or time on the breast and then eliminate and replace with stage one of the stay-and-support approach.

This is the only time I would suggest a dream feed scenario, and only once the other strategy has been implemented.

Lucy Says

Parents should take the overnight module in turns, unless mum has been breastfeeding or is pregnant again or if either parent has a medical condition impacted by sleep deprivation. It is generally a two-person job, so if you are not sharing the load overnight, make sure that you are helping in other ways – getting up early with baby, food preparation, laundry ... Self care of each other continues to be important. If you are parenting alone, make sure you have someone to help out, like a family member or friend – they might not be able to help with the overnight work, but a helping hand with some loads of laundry, a batch of pre-prepared meals, or even just a listening ear can really make a difference.

Chapter 11

Stages to Sleep

W e have started a sleep learning process and you will need to go through stages in order to reach the end goal. We have set the scene, but we can't stay beside the cot or the bed for ever, as this on its own may start to be the problem. I often meet families who are stuck in what I describe as the first phase of sleep learning. They are beside the cot implementing a 'shush pat' approach or the widely used 'pick up, put down' strategy and they are stuck there. Very possibly sleep is not improving either.

Lucy Says

Generally, in order to continue to make progress and initiate a transition away from parental input, we will need to start phasing the parent out of the room, as the child starts to feel safer and more secure in the overall context of their sleep, so I will walk you through the stages.

Stage 1: Nights 1–4

At bedtime

For the first four nights, stay beside the cot or bed, down on the floor ideally, at your child's level. Avoid sitting on a stool or the end of a bed; be low down in an effort to prevent standing or sitting. If the cot is still at the mid-level position and the child is not yet mobile, you can sit on a stool or chair.

As described at the start, use the stay-and-support settling techniques outlined – physically, verbally and emotionally attending to your child. But as the first few nights pass, I would encourage you to do less – less touching, less talking, less intervention – so that you are further weakening the input needed and avoid creating new or additional sleep associations.

Lucy Says

When you begin the first night you may never envisage that doing less is a possibility, but this is a symbiotic relationship – the less you do, the less they will need – and your child will start to feel confident without as much support from you. Don't forget, they are designed to do this; you just need to create the space!

If you continue to over-help as the first few night go by, doing too much may make your child cry more as you move away from the cot in the following nights, so consciously pull back once the first one or two nights are under your belt.

If your older child refuses to stay in the bed, continues to get out, tries to sit on you, hug you or even escape from the room, you will need to manage this situation. Most children will stay in the bed, as long as you sit beside them. They may not be happy about the change from, perhaps, lying in the bed with them, or if you take away a drink, but either way they want you to stay.

If they don't respond well and refuse to stay in the bed, then I would use your presence as a bargaining tool – ask them to stay in the bed and if they don't, you won't stay: count to three and then if they have not performed as desired, leave the room. Wait outside the room, count to 10 in your head, then return to the room and escort them back into bed. If they follow you out, return them to the bed and continue. You may need to repeat this exercise on multiple occasions until they respond accordingly, but they will do as requested because they *want* you to be present, even if the terms have changed.

Overnight

Overnight, when your child wakes, respond immediately when you hear them, return to the bedtime position and repeat this exercise in line with the decisions that you have made about the nighttime feeds and other changes you are making. This becomes your new default approach to weaken the cycle of waking.

If your older child comes into your bedroom, immediately get out of bed, escort them back to their bed and repeat. On the return, 'herd' them back, avoid touching or holding or lifting them into the bed; make them do the hard work themselves and encourage them to pull the covers up too, so that you are helping them to become independent of you.

If they need the bathroom, escort them, don't talk and turn away from them while they are busy, so that you don't ingrain unnecessary nighttime activity.

Stage 2: Nights 5–7

At bedtime

Now move to the middle of the room – lie down or sit on the chair or cushion you have been using, somewhere between the cot/bed and the door, where they can still see and hear you. Even if the room is not that big, just move slightly further away from where you started.

- Do your bedtime routine as normal, but then position yourself further away from the cot or bed as appropriate.
- You can still reassure your child using the initial strategy, but more remotely. Continue to prompt verbally and always go over to physically reassure – spend no more than 30 seconds to one minute beside the cot and then return to your new position, so that ultimately they fall asleep with you a little bit further away.
- If you are spending more time at the cot-side than in your new position, you are possibly doing too much and your child may become hysterical as you move further out of the room. Be there for them, relying more on your verbal reassurance than touch. Pat the mattress rather than your child.
- In this case, less is more.
- If the child is more upset than you would like, you can (reluctantly) return to being beside the cot, but you need to practise doing less of everything so that moving becomes a possibility in another night or two.

Your older child may struggle with this element now, and if this happens and they start to get out of bed, you will need to use your presence as a bargaining tool – repeat the process of leaving the room and counting to 10 as many times as necessary.

If you feel that you are not making progress, you may need to decide to go back to Stage 1 for a bit longer and help them learn to stay in the bed and continue to establish the new bedtime. Alternatively, you may need to decide whether they really are bed-ready, bearing in mind that close to three years old is the age at which they can follow intructions and see them through.

Overnight

Overnight, when your child wakes, give them a couple of minutes before you respond. They may surprise you and go back without you. If they do not, return to your position and repeat the exercise. Your night feeds will now be over, if applicable, so you will repeat the stay-and-support approach as necessary.

If your older child comes into your bedroom, immediately get out of bed, escort them back to their bed and repeat. On the return, 'herd' them back, as before.

Lucy Says

You may find that at bedtime the transition is unacceptable and overnight you still need to be beside the cot or bed. Do this in the short term, but keep in mind that you will definitely try to catch up by night 8 onwards.

Stage 3: Nights 8–10

At bedtime

Change your position to next to the door, still lying down, still inside the room but further away, but where your child can *see and hear you*. If this is not possible, for these days of the process your child should still be able to see you, so consider moving to a position further away, but not near the door – this will depend on the layout of the room. Do *not* move the cot or bed once the process has started; only ever change *your* position.

- Continue as you have been, really scaling down the amount of intervention.
- If you have been singing to your child, now is the time to start scaling it back.
- If you have been back and forth to the cot or bed like a yo-yo, then start to pace yourself. Wait two or three minutes or more before you go back over to the cot-side and then return to the doorframe position until your child has gone to sleep.

At this stage I would anticipate that your child is staying in the bed or at the very least only coming out once or twice to test you, but that ultimately you are in control of the bedtime process.

Overnight

Repeat overnight as required. This time, though, start waiting longer before you return to the room; wait for five to seven minutes, as your child's skill of returning to sleep will be emerging. Be careful that when you go to your child overnight you keep touch and conversation to a minimum. If a dummy re-plug is required, do this for a child under eight months; for a child over eight months, put it in their hand and leave.

Lucy Says

Avoid re-plugging the dummy and tucking the blanket or stroking the forehead as this may become an enabler and continue to promote nighttime activity.

Stage 4: Nights 11–13

At bedtime

Move out into the hallway, where your child can still see and hear you, provided light and noise are not an issue. If light is an issue then you will need to either isolate the hallway lighting or pull the door to, to stop the light entering the room and over-stimulating your child. Whether the door is open or closed generally makes no difference, as long as light is not a problem. The door being closed will never be important in this process and we never want to use fear as a motivator.

- Prevent light from the hallway spilling into the bedroom; close all the other bedroom doors and black out the hall window if applicable.
- Do your bedtime routine and then move outside the bedroom. Stand or sit at the door, where your child can see and hear you.
- If you need to re-enter the room, do so on your schedule, not

their demands. Try waiting for four or five minutes to start with, gradually increasing the time. Hum or shush from the door.

- Remain in position until they have gone to sleep.

Overnight

Ideally, overnight wakening will be really diminishing now. If it still happens, return to the room and resume your position, make sure that you wait for five to seven minutes or so before responding. Many parents now know the difference between the cry that indicates that the child will go back to sleep and the one that means they require you for another reason. What you may experience at this stage is a better night, but with an early start. We shall discuss this below.

The older child may still be waking frequently and taking a while to go back. Continue as planned, reducing and removing touch and talk.

Stage 5: Nights 14–16

At bedtime

Move into the hallway; not in view, but where your child can still hear you. Re-enter the room as necessary on a paced basis.

- Move out of view now; take a side step to the left or right or potter around the hallway.
- Go into your bedroom, perhaps put away some laundry, let him or her hear you.
- Return to the doorframe or room if you need to, briefly reassure and leave again.
- If your child understands, tell him you will be back to check on him – and make sure that you do.

Overnight

Repeat overnight as required. Hopefully there won't be, but you may have still some early rising!

Stage 6: Nights 17 and onwards

At bedtime

Come and go as needed over time, working your way downstairs/to the living space, filling up your dishwasher, having a glass of wine or a chocolate bar (my own preference!), observing and listening to your child on the monitor if you are using one.

Overnight

Repeat overnight as required, always giving the child plenty of space to return to sleep. Kids make lots of noise when they sleep overnight, so you may still hear them, but they just don't need you. Now start to look at what you can do to help preserve your sleep – turning down the monitor, closing your bedroom door. If they need you, you will know!

Typical outcomes

Over the first few nights bedtime starts to get easier and better with reduced or no crying. If it is relevant, review timings between bedtime and the final nap, ensuring that the last feed is at least 45 minutes before bedtime and that your child is not getting relaxed on this feed. Extend your bedtime routine and go earlier.

Overnight I would still expect your child to wake and require resettling using your strategy, but if everything is going well as early as night 7 or, more likely, nights 10–14, you will experience less waking, quicker returns to sleep and a more rested child. Continue to review the changes and the timings. Observe the eating structure and milk intake. Make sure that your child is not too cold in the core part of the night.

It may take your child a while to return to sleep overnight with the new approach. It doesn't matter how long it takes, it only matters that they return to sleep with this strategy, thus allowing it to get better and easier.

If you are still using the dummy I would anticipate that the number of times you need to re-plug will shrink over the course of 14 nights so that you are then perhaps experiencing, at most, three re-plugs overnight (normal for a dummy user), with the expectation of improving that in the next month or so.

If you find that your child is not tolerant of you moving away, it may indicate that you have still been doing too much, so return to Stage 1 and see if you can be beside your child while doing very little, so that when you try to move again it is more acceptable.

You may find your child tolerates you going as far as the door, but they are not open to you leaving. This is a tough one to call. For me, it should never be 'sleep at all costs' and you need to decide what you can commit to, just in this moment. If being present is what your child needs, operate in this way for a while and trial leaving at a later date. Obviously if your sleep overnight is improving, then staying is not the worst presentation – and nothing is for ever. The only time it becomes relevant is if the night sleep is not improving. This may mean that your being there at bedtime is still causing the night activity. Staying may be impractical if you have other children who cannot be left unsupervised or for whatever reason it is just not an option for you or your family to stay while this child goes to sleep. If any of these circumstances are relevant, you will just need to power through the upset – ensuring that all the other guides are being implemented as outlined and that you are open to this potential upset at this stage of the process.

Changing the approach – interval visits

Some children find the parent gradually leaving too much to cope with – I describe them as 'all or nothing' kids – and even this over-stimulates them and makes it harder for them to settle. If this is the case, you may need to reconsider whether the stay-and-support is the right approach for your child.

My main objective is to provide parents with an alternative to controlled crying and cry-intensive methods. One of the disadvantages of my approach, though, is that your child may be over-stimulated by your presence. It's a chance I am prepared to take in order for the sleep issues to be managed as gently and sensitively as possible, but it can undermine *some* children's progress. If this is the case for you, you can resort to an interval visit approach as outlined below; but only do this when you have done at least seven days of my primary approach, if you are making an informed choice and you feel it will be best for your particular child.

In this change of approach your child has a few minutes unassisted *without a parent present* so that they learn to soothe independently and so that they are not frustrated by you being there but not doing what you used to.

I suggest that you return to your child at set intervals. Begin with 5 minutes to start with, then 10 minutes and then every 15 minutes until your child falls asleep.

If five minutes feels too long to wait, feel free to start with a smaller waiting period, but be aware that more frequent check-ins may cause more crying. Decide what feels best and stick with that. Be consistent with the time frame you pick; don't wait 10 minutes, and then go back to five or three minutes.

Follow your bedtime routine as outlined with the appropriate timing, put your child into the cot or bed awake, then leave the room.

- Wait for five minutes (or your decided first check-in interval).
- When it is time for your first check-in, go halfway into your child's room – so that they can see and hear you, but not close enough to touch. Say something like: 'Sleep time now, Harry, I'll check on you in a while', 'shush', or your own mantra. Your voice should be positive and loving.
- At the start you can go over to them and touch them briefly, but very quickly. Aim to stop physical intervention and rely more on a verbal and visual visit.
- Leave the room and begin the waiting interval again.
- The second interval will be 10 minutes (or your decided second check-in interval). Check in again using your voice and presence to support your child.

- The third interval, 15 minutes, is the longest you'll have to wait – continue to check in at this interval.
- Repeat the process as long as needed, waiting 15 minutes each time, until your child falls asleep.

Key points for interval visits

☑ Wait the exact interval you've set for your check-ins.

☑ Limit the amount you touch your child; this may tease them and frustrate them further.

☑ Stay just 30 seconds to one minute maximum before you leave again.

☑ If your child cries harder when you check them, you may want to extend your check-in by an additional few minutes.

☑ Watch for sleep cues. If your child is fussing or complaining – not crying or crying intermittently (pausing for more than 30 seconds) – try to wait, even if it is time for a check-in. This is a sign that your child is learning sleep skills and your revisit will likely interrupt the process. If they begin crying once again, start your visits again, using the last interval time you used. For example, if you were to check after 10 minutes but didn't as your child was fussing at the check-in time, but now they're crying again, restart the timer and check in at 10 minutes.

☑ If your child wakes during the night, begin the process again, starting with the first interval.

☑ If your child is sitting or standing when you enter the room, put them down once after the second interval visit.

This approach is most certainly potentially a more cry-intense approach on paper and not a first choice for me as practitioner, but it suits some children better. It may seem more aggressive, but that's not necessarily the case when you swap from the initial gradual retreat as outlined. Obviously, don't do anything you are not happy with.

Early rising

It is likely that your nights are improving. You may, however, start seeing some early waking; for example, your child is sleeping through quite well, but then waking early and either not going back to sleep, or only going back to sleep for a short time and waking again. This *is* part of the process and the part that many families find really hard. *It will pass.* Generally, by the end of the third week you will start to see this fade away; your child will start to sleep until closer to 6 a.m. or beyond, or they wake and return to sleep on their own. Some families may continue to struggle beyond this time frame – the time around 5 a.m. is a very fragile period for sleep.

Commonly, early rising, along with establishing the second nap, is hard to master. It is very much part of the sleep learning curve, with 5 a.m. onwards being the last sleep cycle and the hardest one to complete, and as a result it takes time to land. Be patient – you are very nearly there.

Don't:
- Start reintroducing a night or early morning feed.
- Start bringing them into your bed or the spare bed or leaving the room before 6 a.m.
- Give them toys in the cot to play with.

Lucy Says

Either of these activities is only a temporary bandage and may promote the early activity and reawakening expectation, which can lead back to frequent nighttime activity.

Do:
- Continue with the plan until at least 6 a.m. (and not a minute before). Even if we all know they won't return to sleep, go through the motions so that you don't shift the body clock to wake at this time.
- Make sure the room is dark with no external light creeping in.

- Avoid any noises – central heating clicking on, someone in the house using the bathroom, getting up for work (I know this isn't practical, but you get the idea).
- Make sure that they are not hungry. Re-examine the food intake and ensure that dinner is an evening meal.
- Review the room temperature and clothing to make sure that being cold is not a contributory factor.
- Be consistent at this early time. Many families report that after two to three weeks the child does better if they don't go into them until 6 a.m., but you will need to judge your approach.
- Ensure that the gap of wakefulness before bedtime does not exceed the recommended time.
- Provide the bedtime feed at least 45 minutes before bedtime. If this has slipped closer to bedtime, it can also contribute to waking too soon.
- Examine bedtime. If it is too early due to the naps (i.e. 6 p.m.–5 a.m.), then by 5 a.m. they have had enough sleep. Adjust the day forward so that the final nap is later and bedtime is too, but the wake period is still what is suggested in your notes.

Sometimes, despite our best efforts and plugging all the gaps, some children just wake early. They can't get past this sleep junction and it can be frustrating for all involved, but often only time will resolve it, once you have all the other measures in place. Wait six weeks from the time you started before you reach this conclusion. Examine your child's sleep and make sure all the parameters are being observed.

If you have been working effectively on your child's sleep for six weeks or more and early waking is still an issue, you may have to accept that this is as good as it can get for now and there is not always a solution. However, you can apply the following tips.

Control the naps

You can make sure that the first nap is starting close to 9 a.m. or if you are on one nap that it does not start before 12 noon. Many families tell me that because their child is waking early they have to move the routine back earlier, but I would not let that cycle continue as it perpetuates the early waking. Create the routine and keep to it, as it will move you closer to a 6 a.m. wake time.

Wake to sleep

If your child wakes at a certain time every morning, so, let's say 5.05 a.m., you could try the wake to sleep technique, which involves you entering the room about 15 minutes before the usual wake time and gently rousing your child enough to send them back over to the next cycle and potentially skip the early wake. This will play out in one of two ways: it will be effective – so continue for a few days and be delighted with yourself! Or they will wake when you enter the room and then you know this technique is not for you.

Adjust bedtime

Another strategy that you could try after six weeks or more is gradually moving bedtime later in the hope that this will adjust the wake time. This is applicable when the child has had enough sleep (10–10½ hours), but still wakes before 6 a.m. Then move bedtime by five minutes every day to see if you can adjust the cycle. This can work, but sometimes it backfires with a later bedtime and the same wake time meaning that now your child is getting less sleep again. Examine everything and take it from there. Although I hate unfinished business, sometimes early waking and/or short naps are just what your child is able to do for now and as parents we just need to work through it and tolerate this for as long as necessary, knowing that everything passes with time. In the meantime, take it in turns, adjust your own schedule with an earlier bedtime and enjoy that early time with your child – view it as quality time, if you possibly can!

Road blocks

Sickness and teething

Probably the biggest barrier to this process is the child becoming unwell or starting to teethe. Suddenly things can seem to be falling apart, but although some children do test the boundaries during sickness or teething, sleep doesn't generally just fall apart. What to do?

First, assess the situation.

- Is your child uncharacteristically whiney, fussy, clingy or out of sorts? (Working on sleep rarely effects the mood negatively unless they are becoming unwell or starting a development leap.)
- Are they off their food or drink?
- Have they got or had a temperature?
- Did they vomit?
- Do they have a slight cough, cold, runny nose and bleary eyes?
- Do they have a sore bottom, messy nappy, red cheeks, or are they visibly teething?

Any of the above and a few more beside can cause your promising sleep to unravel – sickness and teething can cause resistance to sleep, a return to crying at bedtime, frequent nighttime activity, early rising and short naps. Although you will be disheartened because you are actively working on your child's sleep, don't be: this will pass and your hard work will not go to waste, I assure you.

Decide whether you need to see your GP. None of us want to be the neurotic parent, but trust your instincts – better safe than sorry. It is not unusual for sleep to be the first weak spot, and the sickness itself will not be apparent for another week. I know that if my youngest wakes at 5 a.m., before the week is out we will be at the doctor with some ailment or other. So it will affect progress, but follow my advice and all will not be lost.

Lucy Says

If your child is unwell and/or starts teething during the process, the best thing to do is to pause, but not regress. You don't want to go back where you have come from, so try to hold the crucial pieces together.

Don't:

- Reintroduce nighttime feeds; provide a sippy cup for water to keep your child hydrated
- Bring them back into your bed, if you are undoing this cycle
- Try to keep moving through the process.

Do:

- Pause where you are in the process, but try not to go backwards.
- Keep bedtime in place, move back to Stage 1 if needed, but try not to go back to holding, feeding or rocking.
- Respond as you need to overnight – pick up and hold, sit in a chair, comfort and support, but don't bring them into your bed, especially if weakening bed-sharing has been your goal. Camp out in the room with them and remind yourself that no one sleeps well in the initial stages of sickness.
- Use pain medication and antibiotics as recommended by your GP.
- Hang in there. As soon as they feel better, you will see the initial improvements return.

As soon as you feel your child is better again – my own yardstick is when they're off antibiotics, with restored mood and behaviour, back on their food and all symptoms have gone – you can pick up where you left off. If you went back to Stage 1 of settling, start to move positions again, this time moving every two days to modify the approach. It will mean that the road to sleep takes longer, but you will still get there.

Other barriers

One barrier to this process working may be a parent who, for whatever reason, is not able to be consistent with the approach and treats the plan like an à la carte menu. This can sometimes work out, but more often than not it creates a mixed-message scenario that reinforces the problems rather than solving them. If this is you, try not to beat yourself up. Select the pieces that *you can* commit to and try to prevent giving mixed messages.

If I were to try and find a middle ground for you I might suggest that you continue to keep the bedtime element in place with the adjusted times observed, a formal bedtime routine and going to sleep in the new way. Often it is the night that parents can't see through. So rather than continually trying to resettle overnight, only to always 'give in' and provide a feed or bring them into your bed, give way to this and know that even by addressing bedtime you will decrease your nighttime exposure. Perhaps if over another month or two it is still not satisfactory, try again and this time see it through.

Apart from not being able to follow through, many other elements affect the success of the plan. The largest barriers are when there is uncontrolled or poorly managed reflux, digestive issues, food sensitivities or intolerances, skin irritations, allergies, constipation, iron or mineral deficiencies, for example. Sometimes it is not possible to identify what is causing what. I have seen countless babies with reflux who sleep great once they are medicated correctly and their sleep issues are addressed appropriately; but I have also seen many families whose issues are not under control or even unidentified and as a result the night waking specifically is not resolved. Unfortunately, you may have to begin this process and then keep addressing whether progress is being made in line with your efforts and if not, why not. Multiple night waking that does not resolve after three weeks or so *may* be indicative of an underlying problem and I would encourage you to go to your GP.

Now that you are prepared to address your overnight activity, we can start to work on naps during the day.

Chapter 12

Landing the Nap

B y now you will have realised that naps will feature quite heavily in your young child's life and will do until they are at least three years of age. As your child grows, their daytime sleep pattern will get more organised, but similarly will also go through a number of transitions, from the early days of requiring five or more naps throughout the day to (at around 18 months) only needing one daytime sleep. It is getting through these transitions and maintaining a correct balance between the sleeps that is crucial, and observing my suggested feeding and sleeping balances will help you do exactly that.

Lucy Says

An under-rested child will not sleep well overnight. A well-rested child with the wrong nap balance will not sleep well either!

Once you have started the bedtime process using the stay-and-support approach, if you would like to establish naps in the cot I recommend that you begin with a nap establishment strategy on *the morning after the first night of sleep learning.*

Ultimately, the cot is the best place for your child to sleep in the day. If your child is under two years of age this is a worthwhile exercise and, while I don't dismiss an older child learning to sleep in the cot, it can of course be harder or impossible to achieve and that nap will likely have passed by the time your child is aged three. Also, if your child is in daycare five days a week, it may be too much of an effort, with not enough days in a row to practise at home; and your priority may be just making sure that your child naps at the right time and gets enough sleep, rather than worrying about *where* the nap happens.

The decision lies with you, but I strongly encourage this part of the plan, and although *you* may think it is too much change all together, generally children are responsive and the end result is just super.

Lucy Says

What could be better than being able to put your child in the cot in the day for sleep and for you to have time for another child or even yourself? When my children were young I used to work when they napped and it was a good way of balancing things, but of course it's your decision.

Naps in a daycare setting

If your child is in a daycare setting, more than likely the nap is already in a sleeping room, unassisted. Parents are often amazed at what a childcare provider can achieve when they cannot. This is normal – the staff are experienced and typically the child learns how to sleep in a crèche environment, even if they cannot sleep well at home. Sometimes it is the same with eating. Of course, this is not always the case and some children are sleep-resistant or short nappers and need to sleep in a pram or chair. Take heart that when you actively work on your child's sleep, as I have outlined, this can have a positive knock-on effect for poor daycare sleep, although some children will *always* sleep less away from home.

Naps with a childminder

If your child is with a childminder, the best place to sleep in the day is still in a cot in a suitable sleep environment, but this is not always possible, so I would encourage parents to discuss with the childminder what they can commit to and how important the time and amount of sleep in the day are to you and the potential knock-on effect overnight.

Lucy Says

- Plan to establish naps in the cot on the morning after the first night.

- If your child is over two or if you work five days a week, you may want to just focus on naps that happen in any way that works.

- Encourage your childcare providers to have a positive input where day sleep is concerned. They have a big influence on how rested your child is. Don't be afraid of this conversation – everyone will have your child's best interests in mind.

Achieving the nap

- Begin with having your child learn to sleep in the cot with the new approach on the morning after the first night of sleep learning or on the first available morning thereafter.
- Ideally, all naps should be in the cot, apart from the back-up/filler (third or fourth) nap.
- The back-up/filler (third or fourth) nap can be motion-

oriented – in the car/buggy/swing/sling – but not the arms, nursing, bottle-feeding or bed-sharing, once we have started to diminish this need, because this is what we are trying to change.

Lucy Says

You don't need to leave the house for a buggy sleep – you could roll the buggy in a quiet dark room or hall if preferred.

What to do:

- Time the nap according to the age-relevant suggestions and your child's sleep cues.
- If you find your child is harder to read or if there are older siblings who over-stimulate them, you could prepare for the nap 20 minutes before the end of the maximum wake period suggested in your feeding and sleeping balance.
- The room should be as dark as at bedtime. Don't feel that you need to create a different environment for nighttime and day sleep; the body's hormones will do that, so you are in no danger of a 12-hour sleep at midday! But it is important to have a dark room to help you promote the sleep hormone and protect the child's ability to achieve and maintain the nap.
- Provide an abbreviated version of the bedtime routine. It is very important that you prepare your baby for naps as well as bedtime. This is often overlooked by parents attempting daytime sleep, but if you think about it, your child will find it very hard to switch off during the day unless they have been adequately prepared.
- Allocate about 10–15 minutes to your nap time routine. If the routine is too short it will not have the right impact.
- Close the blinds/curtains and dim the lights.
- Follow the same order of events every nap time for continuity.
- Use white noise/music if you like during the pre-sleep ritual.

You could pick one track and put it on repeat, turn it off when your child gets into the cot or leave it on for the duration of the sleep, whichever you prefer.

- Change the nappy, put into the sleeping bag (if using one at bedtime). I often take off jeans or tight clothing, but the child can go into the sleeping bag in their day clothes or with one layer removed – judge for yourself.
- Ensure plenty of physical and eye contact during this time to stimulate the relaxing chemical oxytocin.
- Sing a song or songs, or read your child a story, as at bedtime.
- The aim is to relax your child before you put them into the cot.
- Use the broken record technique, saying the same sentence over and over; 'Sleep time, little one', for example.
- Put your child into the cot, relaxed but awake.
- Position yourself on the floor, just as at bedtime, down at the child's level so that you can easily comfort and support them at this time with the stay-and-support sleep learning approach.
- Both parents (and in time, caregivers) should follow the same sort of naptime routine.

If your child typically naps in the cot and you don't normally stay at nap time and haven't made any significant changes, like removing the dummy or bottle or nursing:

- Walk away as you normally do, provided your child is calm.
- If there is a low-grade protest, continue as normal. If the child is inappropriately upset (this can happen even without significant changes – consider it your journey) return to the room.
- Position yourself on the floor, down at the child's level so that you can easily comfort and support them with the stay-and-support sleep learning approach.

Lucy Says

If you are overwhelmed, forget about the cot; just continue as you used to achieve your naps but at the suggested times. If you generally feed to sleep, don't worry about confusion at nighttime – a different part of the brain controls day sleep – just make the nap happen. If you use a buggy, continue to do this. You can always start with cot naps in a week or two. I don't want you to run out of steam by trying to address all the issues at the same time. This is your journey and ultimately your decision. It will help if you make the space dark for the nap, even if you are doing it somewhere other than the cot. If you prefer, you can work on just one nap. If that is your choice, Nap 1 is the best one to work on; Nap 2 is much harder!

One mum I was working with recently found it depressing doing naps in the cot and wanted to have more flexibility, but she thought she was being selfish. Flexibility can come anyway in time, but if you feel that your emotional well-being is at risk and you don't want to be dictated to by naps, then just make the nap happen and review your progress with this approach to see if the quality of this type of day sleep still helps your child sleep well overnight.

If the nap just isn't working, you can:

- Try for one hour to help your child to take the nap.
- If after one hour this hasn't happened, do the exaggerated wake-up (see page 156) and try again later.
- If a nap attempt has failed, try to have your child calm in the cot before taking them out, after the exaggerated wake-up.
- You will probably have to try again within one hour of the failed attempt. Watch for sleep signals and adjust your feed structure accordingly. The feed can be adjusted to make way for the sleep, in the short term anyway.

Lucy Says

Avoid aborting the mission at the first attempt and going back to your original approach as you may fail to establish naps in the cot by training them to wait!

Try to have your child take a nap in the cot *twice in one day* before you move to a back-up sleep.

Only attempt the nap in the cot twice. Normally, if the first attempt has not worked, the second one will, and naps with the new approach will start to bed in straightaway.

- You may find that the first nap does happen for you but that your child wakes early from the nap. If this happens, when you enter the bedroom, unless you feel that they can be easily returned to sleep, just get them up and move to the next nap period. You can work on this element, if needed, in time.

- If you have tried the cot twice in one day, don't try the cot again. Even if you have had two attempts that did not work, or perhaps two that did but were short, or one that worked and one that didn't, your child will still need more day sleep. I strongly discourage trying the cot again; instead provide a back-up plan – use the car or buggy, sling or swing to achieve the balance of today's sleep and work on this again tomorrow. This way you won't stress your child too much with the cot or the bedroom – or yourself for that matter – and everyone gets a breather. Draw a line underneath today and maintain the bedtime process, and then you can actively begin on the nap again tomorrow.

Lucy Says

As your day unfolds, make sure that you are closing the gap between day sleep and bedtime with back-up or filler naps that are motion-oriented. Don't worry at this early stage about duration of sleep – concentrate on achieving the nap with the new approach.

Try not to worry that the day sleep in the cot is finished early, that the lunch time is super early and that there is a long day to get through. Next week, when this element is a bit more established, you can even this out – for now we can only do so much!

Ensure that your daytime sleep efforts finish in line with the age-relevant daytime suggestions. If the naps are finished too early in the day with no time for another nap, *bring forward your child's bedtime* by adjusting the dinner and bedtime feed and, in turn, the bedtime process by one hour.

Lucy Says

Don't be afraid of a 6 p.m. bedtime – it's not a long-term strategy, but an excellent short-term one to prevent overtiredness, eliminate unnecessary waking early in the evening and possibly a long wake period overnight. It also limits the stress and potential upset that may ensue from being too tired at bedtime and trying to learn a new skill. Don't worry about the wake time either; that will settle down over the next few weeks.

Nap troubleshooting

It goes without saying that, leaving aside of the debilitating effect that broken nighttime sleep can have on the whole family, trying to help a young child nap well is a significant challenge. There is a process to adhere to and it really can take two or three weeks for naps to become established, sometimes even longer if your child is still very young. Remember that nap rhythms may not become established until the child is six months plus; sometimes long naps do not emerge until 12 months, with a small percentage of children only ever catnapping! It's only when you attempt to make changes that you know what your child is capable of. We assume at the start that *most* children need close to the recommended amounts and we will need to achieve that as best as we can. Typically it will be easier to establish Nap 1 and more time-consuming to establish Nap 2, but it will come – and it will be worth the effort!

Lucy Says

At the start, don't worry about the duration of the nap. Towards the end of the second week, if the longer nap is not naturally emerging, you can start to see if you can 'make' it happen – see 'Naps continue to be short' below.

Failed nap attempts

If you keep having a failed nap attempt and/or your child is still crying, this is probably either a timing issue or a lack of preparation before the nap, or both. Normally it's because the nap is too late, so try making it earlier. If not, it may well be going too early – watch their sleep cues and see can if you can land the sweet spot. You may find that initially a short wake period is effective but as your child starts to sleep better overnight, some may be able to stay awake longer between waking and napping, so adjust accordingly.

Not providing a long enough wind-down may also contribute to this, so make sure that you are providing at least 10 minutes, and extend this further if you are having trouble. Ensure that:

- ☑ The room is dark
- ☑ The room is warm enough

☑ There are no loud or sudden noises

☑ If there's music playing, it's not turned off mid-nap

☑ The child isn't overtired before the nap

☑ There's no feed too close to sleep.

Your child appears anxious

Room anxiety can happen as you begin. Everything we are doing is designed to prevent this, but you need to be aware of your child's emotions during the process. First ensure that you are not attempting the nap more than twice in the cot. Second, increase the amount of non-sleep time you spend in the room and extend the length of your wind-down by an extra 10 minutes.

Naps continue to be short

In the first week, don't worry about nap duration. Very often, the nap will naturally get longer, so give your baby a chance, without stressing them or yourself out. Continue to ensure that the room is dark, warm enough and that they are not hungry. Assess the feeding timetable, make sure you are providing breakfast and lunch as outlined and avoid feeding immediately on waking up from a short nap.

As you commence the second week, if Nap 1 is under 45 minutes or Nap 2 under one hour, you could start to lengthen the nap by spending another 30–40 minutes at Stage 1 trying to resettle them. You will need to judge this approach. If within one week you are successful 50 per cent of the time, even if it is only an extra 10 minutes of nap sleep, then continue with this and within another week mid-nap waking will likely stop and a longer nap emerge. If you are having no success, stop trying after the first week and reassess – consider the timing and make sure that overtiredness is not causing this short nap presentation or that bedtime is slipping late again; both reasons for the short nap. Or it may be that this is as well as your child can do for now and things will improve with time.

Naps start and finish early

If naps start early in the day and finish early, this leaves a big gap or brings bedtime forward, so you need to 'calibrate' the day. After 8 to 12 days of starting the plan, I anticipate that if you are applying all my strategies with precision you may also be starting to see some sleeping through the nights, easier bedtimes and nap times, but you now need to adjust the schedule to eliminate the need for the back-up nap when no longer age-appropriate beyond eight months and/or weaken the need for a super-early 6 p.m. bedtime.

This may seem contradictory – we're overriding some of the earlier information in this book in order to streamline the day. I expect Nap 1 to be getting easy to achieve and that you will have started moving away from the cot-side and your input is becoming less needed. Now that is happening, you need to move Nap 1, especially if it is happening around or before 8 a.m. This normally coincides with your child waking early – either around or before 6 a.m. It's very much part of the process, but you need to manipulate things a bit here to make the day run better.

So for the first time I want you to forget about tired signals and concentrate on a time on the clock – you *need* that first nap to happen closer to or after 9 a.m., despite the early wake time – so begin moving the start time of the nap. Move it by five minutes every day until you are closer to 9 a.m. Only back track if your child starts to resist the nap or if the naps starts becoming shorter – this indicates that we've pushed too hard, so reverse and try again in a few days. You may find that your child is just too tired to move beyond 8.25 a.m. or so, but don't worry – rest there for a while and try again in a week or so.

This movement nudges the rest of the daytime sleep later. If necessary, make the same adjustment between Nap 1 and Nap 2, but normally moving Nap 1 is enough. The overall effect is that by starting Nap 1 later, everything else gets adjusted to 30 minutes to an hour later and now the timings are more convenient for all.

ℒucy ℒays

My ideal is that at the end of the process Nap 1 starts around 9–9.30 a.m., Nap 2 around 1–1.30 p.m., and naps finish (once the child is eight months plus) around 3–3.30 p.m. to protect bedtime.

Naps are just not happening in the cot

It happens. Perhaps your child is just not ready or this is not the right time for this exercise or you do not have enough days in a row to practise. If you have been at it for at least one week, abort mission and go back to another way of day sleep. Keep the timings, the bedtime routine before the nap and the dark environment and perhaps take a break for a while – or for ever, depending on your mindset. It's more important that the nap happens than where it happens, and if you have tried and failed, perhaps it is not your time. You can revisit at another stage when you are not coming from a weak position and when your child is routinely sleeping better overnight. Don't give up too soon, but don't bang your head against a wall either! You can always try again at another time.

Chapter 13

Sleep Management

As I get close to completing my work with a family, parents are feeling more confident about their child's sleep and they start to think about the future. Common questions are: How long do I need to continue to prioritise my child's sleep? Can my child have a nap in the buggy? What about days out or travelling? Oh, what happens when the clocks go forward? So I thought that you would like to know as well!

To summarise, I think that you should always put your child's sleep first, but I appreciate that there may be some elements of your life that you have temporarily put on hold while you have been establishing better sleep for your family – and I hope it has been worth it! Obviously I am always going to recommend best practice and that means endeavouring to get your child their recommended amount of sleep, at the right time and in a suitable sleep environment. But you also have to make this work within the fabric of your lifestyle, too. You can be flexible, but not so much so that your sleep becomes compromised and you start to slip backwards. Regressions will happen due to developmental milestones, teething and sickness, transitions through naps and different caregivers, for example, and you can't prevent them happening, but regressions due to an ad hoc approach to sleep can be prevented. In short, positive sleep needs upkeep and maintenance. I normally suggest that 80 per cent of the time you observe best practice, with 20 per cent flexibility for naps on the go and out and about, and bedtime being pushed later.

Lucy Says

Avoid too many days in a row of late bedtimes and missed naps. Then always help prevent a tired cycle from developing with a few early bedtimes.

How do I manage travelling?

In the run-up to any travelling or change in schedule, try to make sure that your child is optimally rested. A better rested child will be much more adaptable than one who is coping with less or frequently disturbed sleep.

Plan ahead:

- If you will be driving long distances, try to ensure that you preserve sleep patterns as much as possible. It can be a good idea to plan your journey to coincide with the first nap of the day so that your child will (hopefully) sleep and then you can arrive at your destination before the second nap of the day.
- If your journey is long, plan to make stops on the way to break the journey up and keep your child from becoming bored and irritable.
- Many parents plan their journey at night and arrive at the destination with their children asleep in the car. If you do this, make sure that on arrival you put your child to bed immediately, even if they appear wakeful. Repeat your bedtime routine and avoid disrupting their body clock by having them awake at night when they wouldn't normally be.
- If you are staying away from home, try to make sure that you maintain your typical bedtime as much as possible. If your

child has their own room at home, it would be great if this could be replicated away from home. Of course, that is not always possible, so if you are room-sharing when you don't normally, move the cot as far away from the family bed as possible in an effort to minimise disruption.

- Bring familiar items from home, such as bedding and sleepwear. It is helpful to bring bedding that has already been used so that your child will be able to smell their familiar sleep environment in the different house. If you use recordings of lullabies, music or white noise at home, don't forget to bring them with you!

- You may find that your baby is unsettled initially in a different environment. Provide plenty of reassurance and encouragement, especially at bedtime. However, avoid making decisions that may have long-term implications: if you don't normally stay with your child at bedtime or perhaps bed-share, be very careful about starting a habit you may not want to keep up when you get home.

- Make informed decisions about staying up late: this will depend on your child's temperament and how they cope with an unregulated day and loss of sleep. Parents of children who manage well can sail through this much more easily than those with a child who becomes fussy and cranky due to lack of sleep. Lost sleep often means frequent nighttime waking and early rising, so beware!

- If you have a late night, resist the urge to allow your child to sleep in – this may make for an unsettled child come bedtime the next night. Try to wake by 7.30 a.m. to maintain the day's timetable. Instead of sleeping in, bring forward the start time and allow a longer duration for Nap 1. Don't be afraid of heading for a nap within an hour of waking up if your child is visibly tired.

- Avoid too many late nights in a row. The aftermath may take many weeks to correct and the fun of the travels may be a distant memory while sleep issues linger.

- Try to make sure that the people around you understand why you are prioritising your child's sleep health and get them involved in the bedtime and nap routines so that they can feel part of the process.

What should I do when the clocks change?

When the clocks go forward in spring and back in autumn, it is a time of transition. It can take a few days, as long as a week, for the child's body to adjust to a different mood lighting caused by losing or gaining an hour and the fact that the natural body clock is being challenged.

I tend to encourage parents not to over-think this transition – as parents we have quite enough to contend with as it is. The best options are the following.

First, ensure that your child is well rested – getting good naps and nighttime sleep – in the run-up to the weekend when the clocks change. Then either:

1. Do nothing; just slot them into the new time. Adjust your clock to reflect the new time and follow your typical daily routine, adjusting feed and nap times, with everything pushed ahead or moved earlier by one hour. Your child will either lose an hour or gain an hour, which means that bedtime is a whole hour earlier or later than the night before. You may encounter a struggle due to the child being undertired or overtired, so respond accordingly as they process the change.

Or:

2. I like to split the difference between the new time and the 'old' time for the first few days, with the notion of getting back to your original bedtime after that. Match your feeding schedule to this change. This way you may alleviate the struggle and allow the child's body to adjust with minimum upset to your daily routine.

Or:

3. If you find that it takes your child ages to adjust, you could consider bringing timings forward (spring) or moving them back (winter) from the Wednesday before the time change. Adjust bedtime to 15 minutes earlier/later on the Wednesday evening before the clocks change and follow this through over the next few days, gradually changing nap times, meal times and of course bedtime by 15 minutes, so that by Sunday you will already be on the correct body clock.

Some important points to remember:

- Decide which option suits you and your child/ren best.
- Continue to pay attention to your child's tired signals and act accordingly.
- Ensure that the room is dark enough at both bedtime and on wake up and also for naps. Use blackout blinds, if you are not already doing so.
- Be flexible. It takes a good few days for our bodies to adjust to the change; that applies to adults as well as children.
- Have a consistent response if they are struggling to sleep and avoid ingraining habits that you may need to address in the future.

What about sleep regression and growth spurts?

It goes without saying that sleep can be frustrating, especially within the first year of life. No sooner do you think that you have established a healthy sleeping pattern then something knocks you off course, from nap transitions to weaning onto solid food, dropping nighttime feeds and, of course, sleep regressions and growth spurts. Many clients ask me if sleep regression is a myth. I can confirm that sleep regressions are indeed very real and can make your child's sleep and, indeed, your own sleep fall apart in a heartbeat with frustrating night awakenings and nap resistance.

The most notable sleep regressions may be observed at 4 months, 6 months, 8 months and/or 9 to 10 months, 12 months, 18 months and 2 years. You will be pleased to know that not all families will experience a regression at each of these intervals, but you may find that one or two of the regression phases are more disruptive than the others.

At six months, parents will often observe a distinct deterioration of their child's sleeping pattern and, regrettably, these changes are often permanent, as mentioned in the earlier chapters of this book. This regression may mean that you experience very frequent night arousals that require your assistance to help your child back to sleep. It is at this point that parents may find they are re-plugging the dummy more times than they can count or perhaps feeding times occur more frequently. If to date you have created a parental dependency, such as nursing, feeding or rocking, to enable your child to go to sleep, this may mean that within a few weeks you may have to establish a new way of helping your baby go to sleep at bedtime, if the fractured sleep phase continues. You can work through the stages I have detailed in this book.

Most regressions can last from two to six weeks. Older children, if healthy sleep habits have already been established, will likely go back to sleeping through and napping well once their brain has processed the developmental changes. At six months this may not be the case and it is not so much a regression as a signal of the new way your child is going to sleep. Unfortunately, you may have to weaken any co-dependency when falling asleep, structure your night feeds and establish a predictable layout to your day – refer to previous chapters to achieve this.

To survive a sleep regression without causing further sleep damage, consider the following.

1. Offer additional feeds. Sleep regressions and growth spurts can often accompany each other. Don't be nervous about offering extra feeds, both at night and/or during the day, during this tricky time. It is a temporary approach but necessary to ensure that you are meeting your child's needs.

2. Provide more reassurance, comfort and support. Add extra time to your bedtime routine and be as responsive as you can without creating nursing or holding sleep associations.

3. Be sure that you are not allowing your child to become overtired. Don't keep times the same if sleep is interrupted; bring nap times and bedtimes forward and try to avoid overtiredness.

4. Draft in support – share the load. Even if mum is still on maternity leave, take night duty in turns. Ask for help from friends and family so that you continue to look after yourself. You are no good to baby if you are worn out.

Growth spurts and sleep regressions are not the same thing. The sleep regression is largely due to significant mental and physical development, whereas the growth spurt is due to gaining weight and growth. Typically you may experience a growth spurt around 7–10 days; 2 weeks; 4 weeks; 8 weeks; 12 weeks; 4 months; 6 months; 9 months; 11 months; and 12½ months.

You will be pleased to hear that, just like the sleep regression, your child may not experience all of these. You may even find that sleep improves during this stage. Sleep regressions and growth spurts often overlap, but they are not the same. A growth spurt will likely last three to seven days, but a sleep regression up to six weeks. I would typically want parents to have an existing problem for four weeks before we would start to consider it a sleep issue that requires intervention. Generally, if healthy sleep habits have been already formed by practising my approach, they will re-emerge within this time frame.

Be careful that you don't attribute all of your sleep issues to regressions, growth spurts and teething. One month of sleep issues plus fractured sleep and continuous short naps indicate a larger sleep disorder that ideally should be examined and worked on to improve sleep for all the family.

What about nightmares and night terrors?

Sleep disturbances are a normal part of development, but they can be difficult for the parents and sometimes the child. We all go through various stages of sleep during the night and have 'partial arousals', where we wake momentarily but immediately go back to sleep. It is at this point that some children can become susceptible to sleep disturbances such as night terrors, sleep walking and sleep talking. Sleep disturbances of this nature tend to emerge beyond the age of two and also seem to affect boys more than girls. It is important to note that if your child is experiencing any of these it is not a sign of a serious emotional disorder, but typically manifestations of a developing neurological system. Nightmares and night terrors are compounded by not getting enough sleep, so ensuring that your child gets as much sleep as possible will definitely help.

Nightmares

Nightmares are a normal part of development and happen during the second part of the night during REM or dreaming sleep. It is a very common complaint, especially between the ages of three and six years, with some studies suggesting that a quarter of all children have at least one nightmare per week.

A nightmare can be very alarming for a young child and the fear is very real: they most often dream of being chased or trapped. Your child will typically call for you or come into your bedroom looking for reassurance and comfort; which you should provide. It can be useful to avoid allowing your child to be exposed to scary or frightening images, programmes or sounds. Carefully pick the type of books that are read at bedtime and be mindful of anything that may cause fear and anxiety. Talk to your child about what disturbs them, ideally during the day, and consider a coping mechanism for scary thoughts; perhaps a monster spray, a magic wand or shield or a special stuffed toy to keep the child safe.

Ideas that can help:

- If you are open to it, have the family pet share the room with your child.
- Have siblings share the room, as long as they behave!
- Ensure that your child is relaxed ahead of bedtime, avoiding stimulating activity, televisions and computer games.
- Be mindful of what your child is seeing and hearing to avoid anxiety.

Night terrors

Night terrors are easily identified and typically happen within the first few hours of sleep, during deep non-REM sleep. During an episode the child jolts awake from deep sleep, eyes wide, frightened, screaming/shouting and possibly sweating, with a racing heart. As this is a partial arousal disorder, your child is not awake, will not recognise you or realise you are there and may push you away while at the same time call for you. Unfortunately this can last for up to 15 minutes and then end suddenly. Your child usually won't even remember having the night terror. It can be very upsetting for us parents to witness children so distressed; but they are not symptomatic of a psychological disorder.

Commonly night terrors will happen within two hours of the onset of sleep. While some may happen throughout the night and/or the early part of the morning, this is extreme and commonly indicates a child who is not efficient at sleeping independently.

The single biggest cause of night terrors is being overtired, so ensuring that your child gets enough sleep can in some instances diminish significantly and sometimes completely eliminate the phenomenon. As little as an extra 30 minutes of sleep at the start of the night can make all the difference.

- Don't try to wake your child. There is no benefit for them to be roused and they may be more upset on waking up, as they are not actually awake during the night terror.
- Avoid touching or picking up your child – this can sometimes prolong the terror – but sometimes singing gently can help.

- Ensure that your child is safe and cannot come to harm if they are thrashing about.
- After the episode, guide your child back to bed.
- Stay with your child and reassure them afterwards until they are calm/have gone back to sleep.
- Avoid discussing the night terror in the morning, as your child will not remember the event.
- Consider an earlier bedtime and ensure that you have regular sleep and wake-up times for every day of the week.
- If the night terrors are happening regularly, keep a sleep diary in an effort to see a pattern. If they are happening at the same time, you can try to pre-empt the partial arousal by gently rousing your child 15 minutes before the episode typically happens – just enough to make them roll over and mumble, for example, and then go back to sleep. When this is implemented for up to 10 nights, it may help to break the cycle.

If you are in any doubt about your child's sleep disturbances it is advisable to seek medical advice.

Nightmares vs night terrors – knowing the difference

Nightmares	Night terrors
A scary dream during REM sleep, typically during the second half of the night	A partial arousal during non-REM sleep, within the first few hours of sleep
Child may be frightened and anxious afterwards	Child will be calm after the event
Child may be hard to settle after the nightmare	Child falls asleep easily after the event
Parental reassurance and comfort required	Parents should limit physical and verbal support
Child will remember the nightmare in the morning	Child will not recall the episode

How do I make room-sharing work?

Having two or more children share a room can be a sleep challenge for some parents. The first key guideline is to ensure that all parties who share a room must be able to sleep through the night. If you have multiples, you must have your child or children learn to sleep through the night in the same space, without panicking and hooking out a wakeful child in an effort to preserve the sleep of another. My ideal scenario with siblings is to have them independent and sleeping well in the overnight period before you put them together. I would sometimes even remove a good sleeper, help the sleepless child learn the skill of consolidated sleep and then reunite them.

After that's taken care of, it is important that you have some room-sharing guidelines for the young children to adhere to, for example: No talking once the lights are out; No waking someone who is already asleep.

It can be helpful to stagger bedtimes in the beginning to avoid over-stimulation in the run-up to bedtime. Obviously, it may take a while for all the parties to get good at sleeping together, but persevere if this is what you want for your children, or of course if space dictates that your children must share.

What happens when I return to work?

Returning to work and easing your baby into a crèche can be a daunting prospect for many families. For some, just the thought of leaving your baby for long periods of time can be difficult enough, without the added challenge of preparing your child to sleep well there too. Lots of the families that I work with share the same concerns and I have put together some helpful strategies and things to think about to make the transition as smooth as possible.

As you will know, achieving enough sleep can be a source of frustration for some families and this can often become heightened when a daycare environment is introduced. To begin, I would encourage you as a family to do your best to ensure that your child is a relatively solid sleeper before you expect them to nap well in another location. Four to six weeks before your return to work, consider if you are currently helping your child to achieve their daytime sleep by holding, rolling or feeding them, which may not be possible for your childcare provider(s). If your child's sleep currently requires a high level of parental input and/or is routinely on the go, consider how that may translate to daycare.

Typically, when your child starts in a crèche, there will be a dedicated sleep room with cots for younger children. This will be where your child is expected to snooze. Generally, the use of bottles and buggies to enable sleep is not encouraged or allowed, so it is a good idea to consider weakening the sleep aids at home first, so that when you hand your little person over, they are already quite skilful at independent sleep. This may still mean that they find it more challenging to sleep in a strange place, potentially with other children, but any ability that is already there will make the transition that bit easier for them. Making sure that your child is well rested before they start in crèche can also be a massive bonus; the more rested your child is, the more flexible and adjustable they will be.

Make sure that the crèche you select offers a sleep-inducing environment – you may be surprised that this is not always a given. Sleeping in a communal environment is another skill that your child must acquire here, and that is more readily acquired if the room itself is sleep-inducing – adequately dark and with limited or masked outside noises and distractions. Many crèches play music during sleep time and while this is not entirely a bad thing, the use of white noise would be better and more conducive to sleep. Either way, music or white noise may help mask external noises and help your child stay asleep. Don't worry about having to use it at home if you don't already; your child can have different associations for different locations and will be able to separate the conditions in the home from those in the childcare environment.

Share with your crèche the daytime schedule you already have. Hopefully they will be accommodating rather than making your child fit in with their own schedule. Collaborate so that your child's needs are prioritised, especially at the start of the transition.

Routinely, your child will be initiated into the crèche environment two to four weeks before they begin their full- or part-time attendance. These social hours are a great way of introducing your child to their new surroundings and caregivers. Ideally, leave the sleep introduction to the later part of the initiation time, so perhaps give it a week or so of going there to play before attempting sleep. The first nap of the day is generally the easiest one to achieve and this can be the best one to start practising with. Always let the staff manage sleep in the new environment. Many parents feel they should show their childcare providers what they do in their own pre-sleep ritual, but I would not encourage this. Explain it to them, but allow the crèche team and your child space to learn what works for them. Remove yourself entirely from the process as this will not be a long- or even a short-term solution. When you hand your child over, make sure you always say goodbye. You probably won't feel happy or confident to start with, but try to be, so that your child doesn't pick up on your anxieties and feel nervous.

As with all transitions, you will need to give it time to bed in. As you do this, avoid your child becoming overtired, which may expose you to nighttime activity. As your child processes the changes and possibly gets less daytime sleep than normal, bring bedtime forward to help pick up the potential deficit and to weaken an overtired cycle, which you really will want to avoid. Don't be surprised if your child is super tired from 6 p.m. onwards; allow earlier sleep at the start and then the later bedtime can be reintroduced when the settling-in period has ... settled in!

What about separation anxiety?

As your child's sense of self starts to emerge within the second half of the first year and their ability to roam and explore independently is more established, separation anxiety can begin to kick in and then fluctuate for the next two years. As sleep is the biggest separation for a child not bed-sharing with the parents, you may experience a resistance to sleep time. You might consider implementing some of the following suggestions.

- Play lots of games that allow your child to develop object permanence. Peek-a-boo, jack in the box, hiding items under a blanket; all of these can help your child to learn that even though they can't see an item, it still exists. This can help them understand that mummy and daddy go away but always come back.
- It is important to always tell your child when you are leaving and to avoid sneaking away from them, even though it can sometimes be hard on both the parent and the child. Stealing away can fuel your child's anxiety around separation and make the problem worse. Practise going away and coming back in your own home if you feel that would help.
- Provide your child with a transitional object like a safe blanket or toy that will help them feel close to you and to help ingrain positive associations with sleep.
- Add extra time to your bedtime routine. Tagging on an extra 5 to 15 minutes can really help to bridge the separation void. Indulge in lots of extra physical and eye contact in the child's bedroom, helping prepare the alert body for sleep.

What about teething?

This is a developmental issue that continues for at least the first two years of life. Some children find teething especially hard and their sleep can often be fragmented due to pain. This stage is often most difficult until the tooth erupts and typically your consistent sleeper will return to sleeping well, until the next time ...

During a teething phase, observe the obvious signs – flushed cheeks, drooling, sore bottom, irregular bowel movements – and be supportive. Provide extra reassurance and even consider having some daytime sleep on the go in the car or the buggy instead of the cot, until the tooth cuts through. Teething episodes also contribute to short naps and interrupted nighttime sleep. Under the guidance of your GP use a pain reliever if appropriate.

Are developmental milestones and sleep disturbances related?

As mobility increases, your child will become more interested in roaming and exploring. You may get the sense that your nine months plus child has better things to do than sleep, and resistance to rest can become relevant. To help with this transition, consider:

- Offering lots of practice of their new skills. Factor in lots of floor time and try to avoid long periods cooped up in the buggy or the car.
- Make a safe place in the home where your child can roam around. At this stage your child needs to maximise movement during wake time, which will alleviate the desire to practise the new skill instead of sleeping.

Expect resistance to wax and wane as the new skill becomes established. As your child becomes more verbal, ensure that you give a clear message where sleep is concerned. Meet objections, don't give in to stalling tactics or to demands about sleeping or refusing to sleep. Some toddlers' favourite phrases are 'No nap' and 'I don't sleep'. Provide lots of choices around sleep, such as which pyjamas they will wear and maybe which two books you will read.

In general, I would encourage parents to be aware that there are many variables that influence your child's sleep patterns, even if they have appropriate sleeping habits. This awareness can help parents to understand sleep regressions and to be confident that, as long as a degree of consistency is maintained, consolidated sleep will return once the stage has passed. Problems that persist beyond four to six weeks may require a modified version of the original approach for your child: you will follow the same process, but go through the stages more quickly.

When to move from two naps to one?

It is usual for the last nap transition – from two naps to one – to happen at around 15–18 months of age. Making this move prematurely can increase the possibility of nighttime sleep issues. Most children perform better with two naps until this slightly later age group. This is your last nap transition and routinely the most challenging. Once again the nap power play may be at work. When your child is ready for one nap it is the second nap that is maintained and the first nap that is retired – although the child may not be a willing participant! To make sure you don't create any difficulties, keep in mind the following:

- When your child is ready for one nap, this sleep should ideally start between 12.30 p.m. and 1 p.m. and be one to two hours plus in duration.
- Maintaining a wakeful period not more than four hours between the nap and bedtime is crucial, so the closer to 1 p.m. this sleep begins, the better.
- Understand that the gap between waking and napping is not the important one; it is the one between the nap end and bedtime that is significant

You will know your child is ready for one nap if:

- They are at least 15 months old and routinely sleep through the night.
- They have resisted either the first or second sleep for a week or more.

If the resistance is to Nap 1, the transition can be easier. You may find that your child wants to be asleep by 11.30 a.m. and allow that to start with; then move the time by 15 minutes every two days until the start time is beyond 12 p.m. and closer to 1 p.m.

If, however, the resistance is Nap 2-oriented, your child may not yet be ready and you may just need to shorten the duration of Nap 1 to 45 minutes or even 30 minutes. Then you will be able to start the changes as above when this approach stops working.

Additionally, most children will nap until they are three years plus. This transition is also fairly organic: the nap either reduces to one or one and a half hours a day until they just stop sleeping; or you may find that the duration stays at around two hours, but they don't nap every day. Even when day sleep is no longer required, a provision for 'quiet time' in its place is a great strategy to help your child switch off and relax after lunch.

How to transition to the big bed?

I recommend keeping toddlers in the cot for as long as possible and don't normally suggest making this transition until around two and half to three years of age. Developmentally, your child then has the mental reasoning necessary to understand words like 'Stay in your bed all night'. Cognitively you want your young child to have some impulse control and that when you issue an instruction to them they not only understand what you are saying but they can also make an effort to comply.

Before making the big move from cot to bed ideally your child would be at least two and a half years old and routinely sleeping through the night. Then it is worth discussing your plans with your toddler and giving them a sense of ownership over their sleeping arrangements. It can sometimes be helpful to give them lots of small choices around their sleep, such as where the bed should go, where they will keep their books and what duvet cover they would like. This transition may also coincide with your plans to toilet train your youngster and you don't want to overload them with lots of changes all at once. It makes sense to transition to the big bed first and then tackle the training – but you know your own child best. It may also coincide with the arrival of a new brother or sister; so you don't want to speed up this transition with rumblings about the cot being required for another little person who may already be treading on your toddler's toes.

Get your small person invested in the new sleep plans, take them shopping to pick out the new bed and bed linen and let them 'help' you organise the bedroom for the new bed.

You will need to amend your existing bedtime routine and make sure that you are firm about the boundaries. Try not to fall into the trap of 'one more story'; these stalling techniques can often spiral out of control. Also, avoid agreeing to stay lying down with your child or holding hands at bedtime, unless you plan to co-sleep or room-share.

I advise that you continue with the structured bedtime routine that, with the exception of the wash/bath/teeth, should happen exclusively in the child's bedroom so that they can have positive associations with sleep. I often use a lamp on a timer to indicate the start and the end of the routine that should happen before they climb into bed. Have a predictable sequence of events that happen over the 20–30 minutes before sleep time. Enjoy this close, one-to-one time with your child and indulge in lots of physical and eye contact and low-key activity such as book reading, storytelling and relaxation exercises.

If at the start your toddler keeps getting out of the bed, calmly return them to the bed and explain, 'It's sleep time now'. If your child is struggling to adjust to the bed, you may have made the change too soon. Don't panic, just put them back in their cot and wait a little longer.

When good sleep turns bad!

Finally, remember that your child's sleep is a work in progress. It requires upkeep and maintenance and refining as they transition through the various stages of childhood. It is not unusual for me to hear from a parent that their dream sleeper has turned into a awful sleeper. My first question will be 'What has changed?', and although the parent may report that nothing has, that will rarely be the case. So I have prepared a list of seven remedies to apply if this should happen to you.

There are many possible reasons, but the most common culprits are:

- Recent sickness or bout of teething
- A holiday
- Nap transitions
- Developmental milestone
- Bedtime that has become too late
- Dropping the dummy

The problems can be initiated by any one of or a combination of these events and, of course, others that I haven't listed, each of which contributes to a cycle of overtiredness and fuels the sleep issues, until sleeping through the night becomes a distant memory. I often describe this scenario as the elements of a perfect storm.

What can you do to get back on track?

1. Change what you do. Forget about what you used to do and have a new plan of action to remedy the situation. The greatest solve-all solution to a large percentage of sleep issues is to bring bedtime forward. When a child is not sleeping, maintaining your original time for sleep adds to the problem. To undo the overtired cycle, significantly adjust the time you start your bedtime routine. Consider your child's mood and behaviour in the early evening. Many parents observe that their child's mood can change between 5 p.m. and 6 p.m. with irritable or even hyper behaviour – even if the child has napped well. This is where going to bed early can help. Aim for your child to be asleep by 7 p.m. – even earlier if they are visibly tired. This is not necessarily a long-term solution, but it can certainly be implemented to correct the current issues. Once they are resolved, bedtime can become later again. Further, don't worry that an early bedtime will encourage an early wake time. To start with, we want to ensure that consolidated, uninterrupted sleep returns to your family unit; sleeping later in the morning can come with time. Also, the early bedtime can often produce a late wake time anyway, so don't let that stop you from implementing the advice.

2. Start the day. Make sure you wake your child in the morning no later than 7–7.30 a.m. Even if they have had very disturbed sleep, allowing them to sleep later will make the problem worse and dig your sleep deprivation hole even deeper. Consider this a corrective phase. Once the problems are fixed you can go back to what you were doing before, but to help change come, you need to change what you do.

3. Re-establish the daytime sleep. Sleep issues feed each other. If your child is under five and not sleeping well at night, consider reintroducing the nap in an effort to help them become better rested. Most children up to the age of three will still biologically require a day sleep, so help it happen. After 18 months a lot of children need just one nap, and the ideal time for that to happen is from 12 noon onwards. If they are resistant to napping in the cot or bed, just help the nap happen in any way possible – car, buggy, couch. If a nap is not achievable, encourage quiet time instead. Make sure that quiet time does not include television but rather reading or listening to audio books, for example.

4. Add extra time to your bedtime routine. Your child may feel that they are not seeing enough of you, or at least getting enough of your undivided time. Bedtime is the perfect time for families to indulge in one-to-one time. Make it work for you where sleep is concerned – be in the bedroom, with the lights low. Make sure that it is non-stimulating and calm. Spend more time than usual in order to correct the issues.

5. Limit the use of electronic media and television. Obviously in the last hour before bedtime, but also through the course of the day. As parents, we can often rely more heavily on gadgets than we would like and routinely their use derails sleep – cutting short the amount of deep, restoring sleep children have and alerting the waking part of the brain when we want it to slow down. It can be challenging to alter our use of devices, but a challenge that can really pay off.

6. Get more active. Spend more time outside, specifically in the morning and after the midday sleep. This can help to regulate sleeping patterns and ensure that children are burning off their excess energy. On its own this strategy may be ineffective, but along with the aforementioned changes it will have positive implications for sleep.

7. Be consistent in how you manage your child's sleep disturbances. Routinely, sleep problems are further exacerbated by how we as parents respond. Try not to operate a 'sometimes' method for sleep, chopping and changing how you respond to your child. Pick an approach and stick with it; go back to the start of the stay-and-support strategy if it would help, and work through the stages again. This way you avoid giving them mixed messages and in turn ingraining unwanted activity.

To conclude, it has been my pleasure and privilege to get you this far with your sleep improvements and I wish you and your family well going forward.

Sweet dreams.

Lucy Wolfe

Index

massage, infant 65
melatonin (sleep hormone) 42, 44, 64
milk feeds 117, 121, 123, 125
Moses basket 55, 56
motion suggestions 54–5
music, use of 46

napping 82, 139–43
  achieving the nap 180–5
  child anxiety 187
  controlling 173
  cot failure 189
  in daycare setting 179–80
  duration of nap 188
  failed attempts 186–7
  transition to one nap 205–6
  troubleshooting 185–9
night feed, retaining 158–9
night-weaning
  regulating feeds 154–6
  single feed 157–8
  weaning multiple feeds 156–7

one-to-one time 41
outdoor activity 21, 64, 85
overnight plan 147–149
overtiredness 12–14, 53, 84
oxytocin 44

pacifier *see* dummy
parent, feeling of failure 3
parental dependency 8–9, 10, 11, 70
  dependency levels 9–11, 28
partial arousal 9–10
percentage of wakefulness approach 11, 61–3, 68
picking up 78–9
play time, connected 41

quality sleep 81
quiet time 83–4

reflux and intolerances 65–9
  and feeding 66
  signs and symptoms 68–9

and sleep 66, 67–8
  sleep planning 67
  sleep positions 67
relaxation exercises 90–2, 95
role play 89
room acclimatisation 32–3
room-sharing, with siblings 23–4
  see also sharing, room/bed
routines 16–17, 129, 145

safe sleep 57–8
  guidelines 49–51
security item 35–6
separation anxiety 202
sharing, room/bed 22–6, 55, 56, 57–8, 200
sickness 176–8
sleep
  amount needed 81
  checklist 88
  clock change 195–6
  disturbances 212
  gentle sleep shaping 4, 47–9
  good sleep to bad 207–10
  issues, common 15–16
  phases, natural 8–11, 17
  plan, getting started 18–21, 73–4
  prioritisation need 19
  readiness 13–15, 52
  regression 194–6
  resistance to 7–8
  safe 57–8
  safety guidelines 49–51
  strategies 86–92
  child involvement in 86, 89
  and travelling 191–3
sleep deprivation 2
sleep environment 41–3, 59
sleep learning
  learning process 3–4, 32
  stages 160–8
  barriers 176–7
  changing approach 168–70
  typical outcomes 167
sleep location 21–31, 41–3, 50, 55–6, 85
sleep log 31

212